W9-BUU-621

THE
MAKEUP
WAKEUP

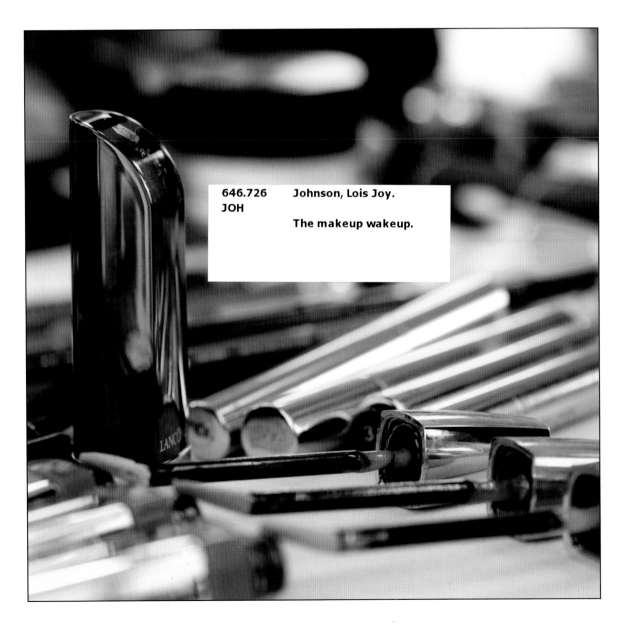

THE MAKEUP WAKEUP

Revitalizing Your Look at Any Age

Lois Joy Johnson and Sandy Linter

Photography by Michael Waring

RUNNING PRESS
PHILADELPHIA · LONDON

Printed in China

9 8 7 6 5
Digit on the right indicates the number of this printing

Library of Congress Control Number: 2010928281

ISBN 978-0-7624-3935-5

Designed by Corinda Cook
Edited by Cindy De La Hoz
Typography: Avenir, Aviano Light, Dorchester, Helvetica Neue,
and Stemple Garamond

Running Press Book Publishers
2300 Chestnut Street
Philadelphia, PA 19103-4371

Visit us on the web!
www.runningpress.com

Page 2: Alva Chinn

Page 6: Karen Bjornson

To our moms, Joan Fuller (Sandy) and Phyllis Wilensky (Lois),
for all those lipsticks, eyeliners, and mascaras we borrowed
that got us started—and, of course, for giving us the love of makeup.

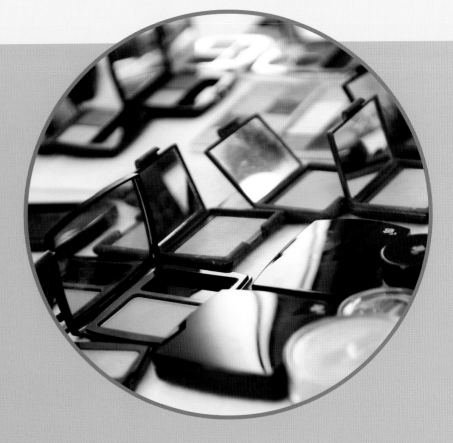

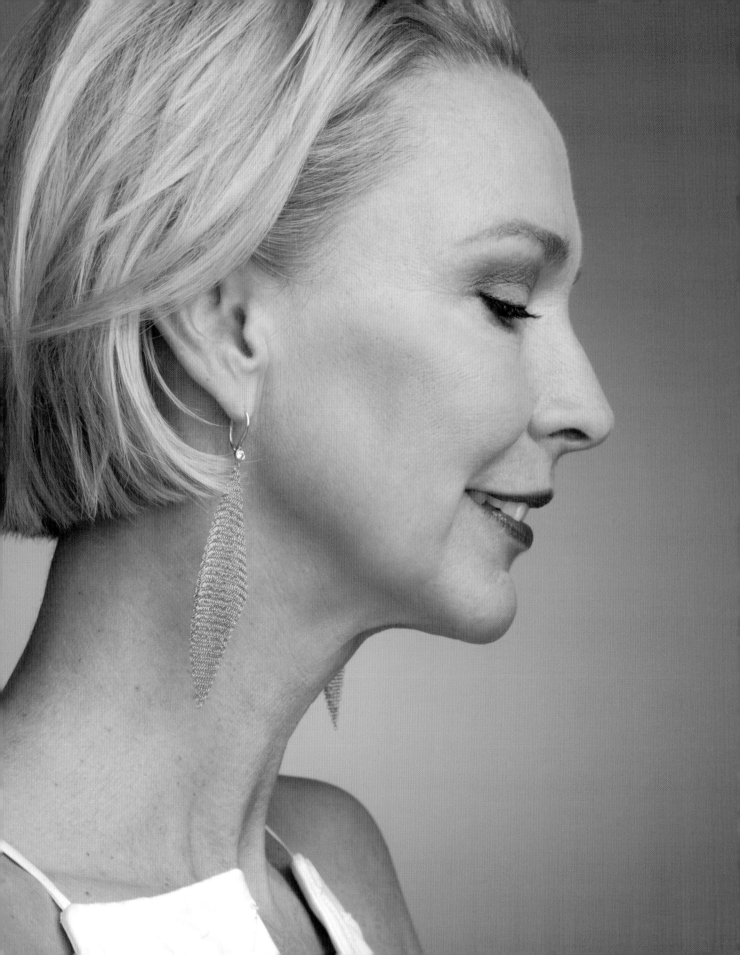

CONTENTS

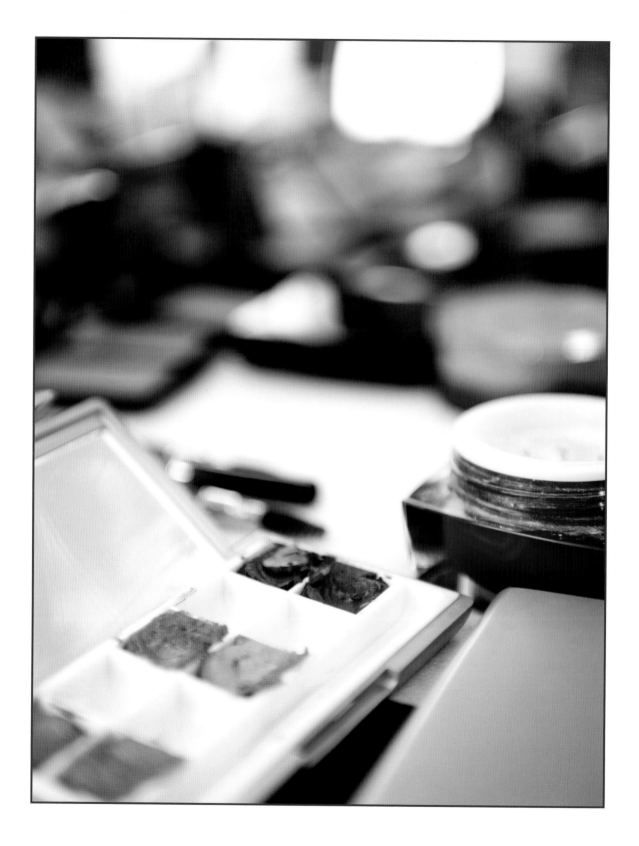

Foreword

Makeup! Maquillage!! Warpaint!!! Who doesn't love it? It's a chance to be creative every day, and by using your face as your canvas, to present yourself as anyone you wish to be. It's a ritual that can be as imaginative and amusing as you like, taking as little or as much time and money as you have to spend. You can pile it on or just curl your lashes, hit your lips with a slash of red, and rush out the door.

I fell in love with makeup as a very young girl in Hawaii at the height of the beehive-and-eyeliner craze of the early '60s. I will never forget the sight of hundreds of kids at my school in Hawaii surrounding a new arrival from California; she was a platinum blonde with an enormous beehive, black eyeliner out to there, and the palest lips anyone had ever seen. Yikes! No one in our little town had seen such an alien, and the race was on to at least approximate her look, by hook or by crook.

Having zero disposable income, there was nothing for me to do but turn to a life of crime. Yes, dear reader, I became a shoplifter—not for long, and not to any great extent, but long enough to be able to transform myself from Mouse to Madame overnight. And Madame wasn't far from the truth, either; after making myself up I looked suspiciously like a very young brothel keeper. Maybe I didn't get the look quite right the first time. But it didn't stop me from trying again and again!

I never really recovered from those early days of experimenting with looks and personas. I still keep up with the new products and colors available every season. All my professional life I have formed strong bonds with makeup artists. They are some of the most magical people I know—determined to transform and beautify the world, one woman at a time.

Sandy and Lois are two of these people. They have figured out what it takes to add glamour, fun, and beauty to every day, and their vast knowledge of products and application makes them the perfect pair to guide those of us who are looking for intelligent answers to the questions of how to present our faces to the world. Their bag of tricks is a full one, and they're willing to share. I love this book as a resource and a roadmap, and I think you will too. Have fun!!!

—Bette Midler

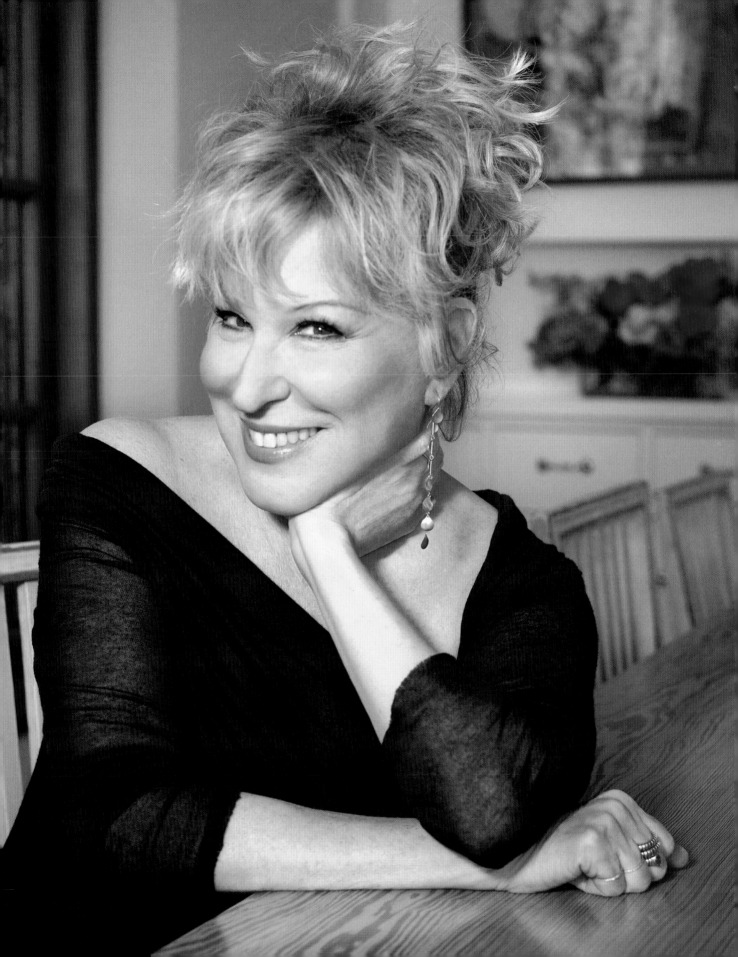

Before

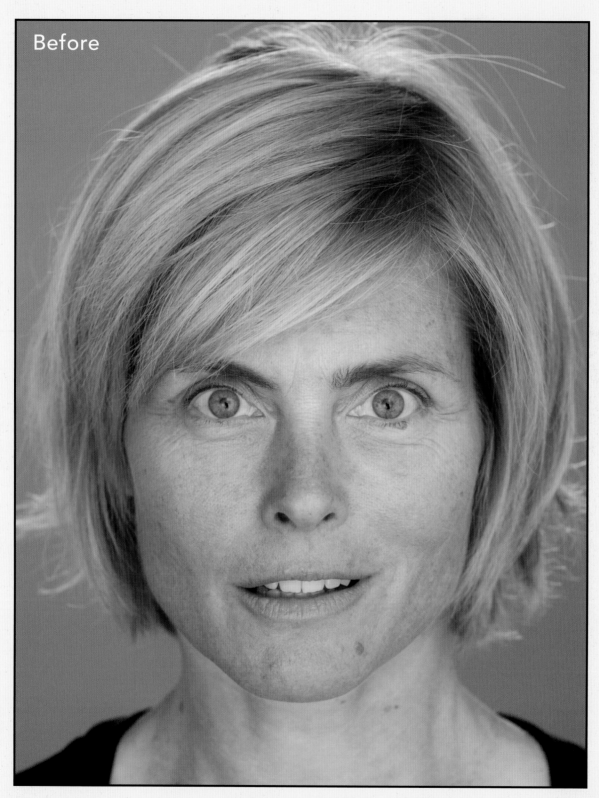

Our cover girl, Kim Alexis

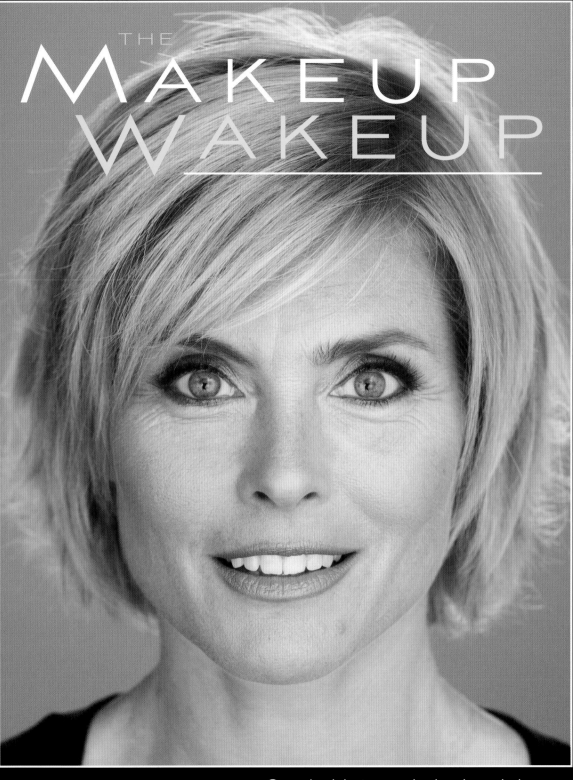

THE
MAKEUP
WAKEUP

Introduction by Sandy Linter + Lois Joy Johnson

After a certain age women hit a beauty rut.

The face you've known and loved has moved on but your makeup hasn't. Makeup tricks that worked in your twenties, thirties, and early forties are letting you down. Every day is hit or miss. You blame your concealer, your foundation, your magnifying mirror, and your BFFs who suggest, "You look tired—maybe you should get your eyes done?" It's an "Uh-oh" moment. Do I need better makeup? Botox? Fillers? Cosmetic surgery? Looking fresh, healthy, and confident is crucial.

Beauty keeps evolving and so do you; beware of holding onto makeup techniques that are actually aging. How do you know that your makeup application has made you look older? When people you love tell you that you look better without makeup. It's time to learn what works at this point in your life. It's time to get serious and rethink your looks. That's where we come in.

We—Sandy + Lois—are, respectively, a celebrity makeup artist and a top beauty editor. We've spent more than two decades working on photo shoots with thousands of smart, accomplished, gutsy women who plan to stay in the game indefinitely. They won't let a few wrinkles or brown spots get in their way and neither should you!

The Makeup Wakeup gives women a new set of options and a brand new way to think about makeup. Face your flaws, then decide whether you'll work with makeup alone or add surgery or a dermatological fix to your cosmetic arsenal. We all age differently and have our own opinions on how far to push the beauty envelope.

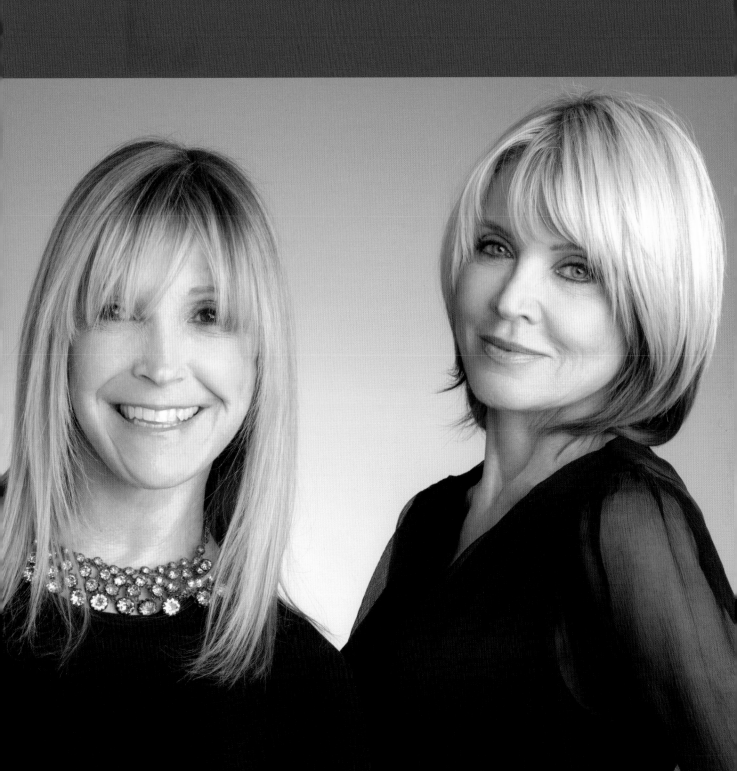

Lois Joy Johnson

Sandy Linter

Use this book three ways.

1

If you want to max out your makeup potential and skip surgery. Makeup alone can make the most of your looks and substitute for (or delay) the scalpel, laser, or syringe. For some women this is enough and we can help you get there. With Sandy's makeup secrets (the same steps she uses on her celebrity clients), plus our product guide, you can look better than ever before.

2

If you want to get the best makeup of your life and decide to mix in some dermatological or surgical options. We reveal how makeup can enhance the solutions offered by Botox, fillers, and surgery. Since we're beauty experts and not doctors, we asked a superstar cosmetic surgeon and two top dermatologists to back us up on the medical advice. Dr. Daniel Baker and dermatologists Dr. Patricia Wexler and Dr. Fredric Brandt—whose clientele lists read like red carpet rosters—provide A-list advice. If you decide "No thanks" on procedures for now, we're there with makeup fixes for every flaw.

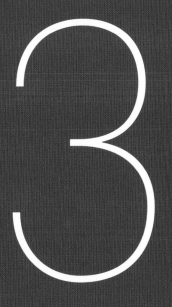

If you're dealing with demons like tanning addiction, hair loss, or menopause pores, there are beauty solutions for every problem. We have the answers to the issues no one talks about but everyone thinks about. If you have a spotty décolletage, skin that acts like it's fifteen instead of fifty-five, or hot flashes that make mush of your makeup, you've come to the right place. Our combination of practical cosmetic and medical advice, and our own "been-there, done-that" attitude, will make a difference.

Get to know us because we're sticking with you.

Lois Joy Johnson is a beauty editor and leading expert on style for women 40+. As one of the founding editors of *More* magazine, she helped launch the Pro-Age Era, working for more than a decade exclusively with models, celebrities, and real women in their forties, fifties, and sixties. Lois has interviewed and photographed hundreds of women who changed the face of beauty and revised our attitudes towards aging. They include Christie Brinkley, Paulina Porizkova, Lauren Hutton, Carol Alt, Isabella Rossellini, Ann Curry, Carolina Herrera, Jamie Lee Curtis, and Diane Keaton. She has been a frequent contributor to *The Today Show*, *The Early Show*, *Extra*, and CNN.

Lois has brown spots, thin lips, really bad brows, and sun damage you wouldn't believe. She's also a natural, low-key make-up, low-maintenance type—and yes, has tons of self-confidence.

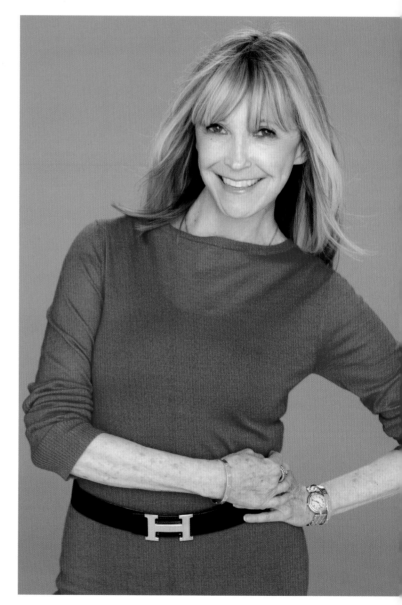

Sandy Linter is a celebrity makeup artist who has inspired the beauty world for more than three decades. Christie Brinkley, Bette Midler, Goldie Hawn, Sigourney Weaver, Katie Couric, Suze Orman, and Martha Stewart are just a few who have experienced her makeup magic.

Sandy's first *Vogue* cover hit newsstands in 1974. Her work has appeared on countless covers since, from *Cosmopolitan* to *Harper's Bazaar* to *More*. She's had the privilege of working with renowned photographers Irving Penn, Albert Watson, Richard Avedon, and Francesco Scavullo; legendary supermodels; world-famous actresses; and even royalty. In addition to her ongoing makeup duties, she serves as Lancôme's Beauty at Every Age Expert.

Sandy, like many of you, worries about her neck. And her face. And other body parts. But, of course, she believes in total makeup, 24/7.

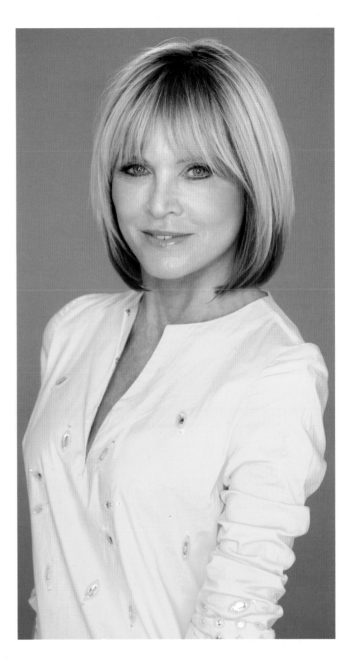

A message about individuality, before we begin . . .

The secret of staying sexy—confidence in doing your own face.
Women age with enormous diversity and feelings about the process. Strong faces with character, interesting features, and a healthy overall look is what we consider beautiful. The women we photographed for this book are women over forty whose integrity, accomplishments, and attitude we admire—and of course their extraordinary beauty and personal approach to aging made them ideal models for us too. It's a very mixed group. From Patti Hansen's fashion-forward spirit and smoky eyes to Karen Bjornson's fine-boned elegance to Lauren Ezersky's edgy approach to Alva Chinn's natural glow and Nancy Donahue's sophisticated, classic style—each and every one of these women is amazing in her own way.

Here's the important part: Each of our sixteen models has her own look, but every single one is facing the camera wearing a variation of Sandy's makeup lessons. The difference is in the level of intensity and choice of color. The steps and techniques remain the same.

Sandy and I worked as a team for years on *More* magazine's annual 40+ Model Search. Thousands of women age forty to sixty-five entered each year hoping to win a modeling contract. Some years as many as 20,000 women sent in their photos and entry forms. These women had two things in common: they had a huge dose of self-confidence and they believed managing their looks was a vital element in achieving their life goals. We can't say it enough. Having control over your looks provides enormous confidence. Being aware of your own looks and how to make them work for you makes confidence sexy.

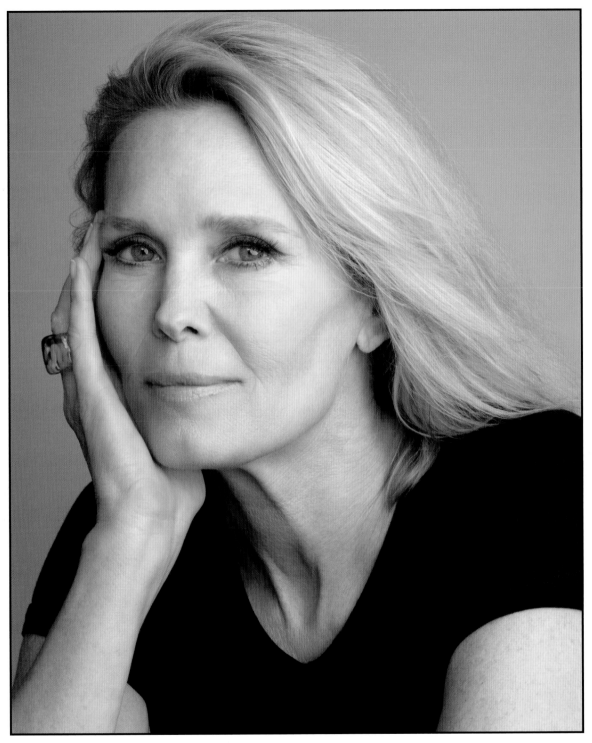

Nancy Donahue

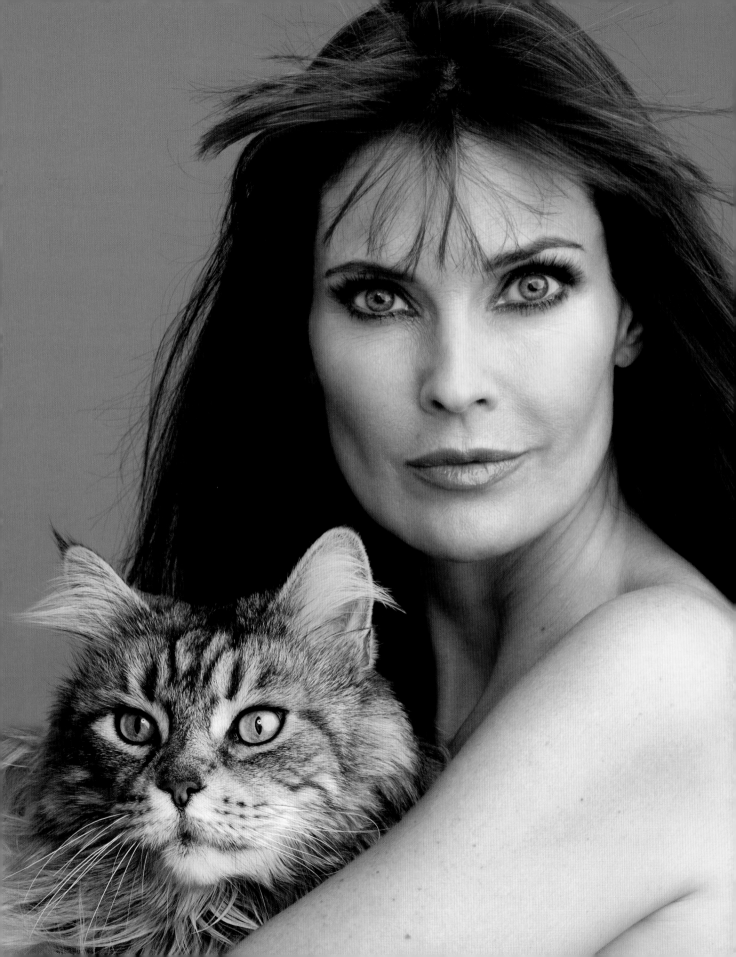

CHAPTER ONE

BIGGER, LIFTED, DEFINED EYES

Think of your face as your homepage . . . Your eyes as your daily blog. Every day they send out new info. If you got three hours of sleep, had a crummy day at work, or drank too much wine with dinner last night, your eyes will tell all. They're the most effective communication tools you have.

Carol Alt

Grown-up Eyes

The problem with our eyes is they change with age and continue to morph no matter what we do. Even if we use $300 eye creams or have plastic surgery, the cumulative effects of gravity, sun damage, genetics, and the loss of collagen and estrogen will stalk us forever. Some of us rely on a routine of Botox and fillers to smooth and fill furrows or minimize bags and circles. Some of us just depend on eye makeup and a pair of sexy sunglasses for age management. We check out our peers and wonder: "Did she get her eyes done? Or is it her makeup?" Because beauty never lets up and we never give up.

Buy and apply makeup for the eyes you have now, not the ones you had ten years ago or even two years ago. Whatever you decide—and you should definitely treat yourself to the best eye makeup of your life—it will change your outlook.

What was I thinking? Or, My Life in Eye Makeup

We've been there with you.

Nothing guarantees self-assurance and a snappy attitude more than eye makeup. We should know. Sandy and I have been wearing eye makeup since junior high, way before our lives led us into the beauty biz. We've been work colleagues for years but I never saw Sandy without makeup until we shot her "before" pictures for this book. She practices what she preaches. See for yourself on page 273, where we wrap up with a makeup lesson To-Do List featuring Sandy herself taking you through the steps.

We think dermatological procedures and eye lifts are great options but here's the untold truth: you will still need eye makeup to finish the job and not your same old eye makeup either.

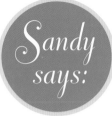

Sandy says: I had my eyes surgically enhanced twice (once at thirty-seven and again at sixty) for practical reasons. Having my eyes done gave me total freedom with my makeup choices and application. Since I find eye makeup the most inspiring of all makeup, surgery eliminated the need to correct or compensate. It just made makeup fun to wear again. My job as a makeup pro is to make other women look beautiful. How could I appear on set looking tired? When my own eye makeup looks great it inspires confidence in my clients. When I make a good visual impression models and actresses relax—they know they're in good hands.

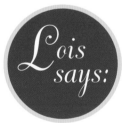

Lois says: As a beauty editor and major makeup cheater I often skip eye makeup and just wear big black Cutler & Gross glasses for definition and style. Frankly, I fell in love again with the whole ritual of liner, foundation, and mascara during the writing of this book. It starts my day with a shot of creativity. I'm all for very strong, clean eye makeup. It makes me feel great even when I'm just working at the computer in jeans.

What the right eye makeup can do for you now

Eye makeup is practical magic. It keeps you from looking washed out and tired, gets you going on a bad day, elevates your mood, and restores your confidence when you don't feel fabulous. It will totally save you when you're having a bad hair day, going on a job interview, attending your college reunion, or meeting new clients for the first time. It will make you feel sexy when you haven't worked out and think you look fat. Eye makeup makes you look polished and gives your face definition.

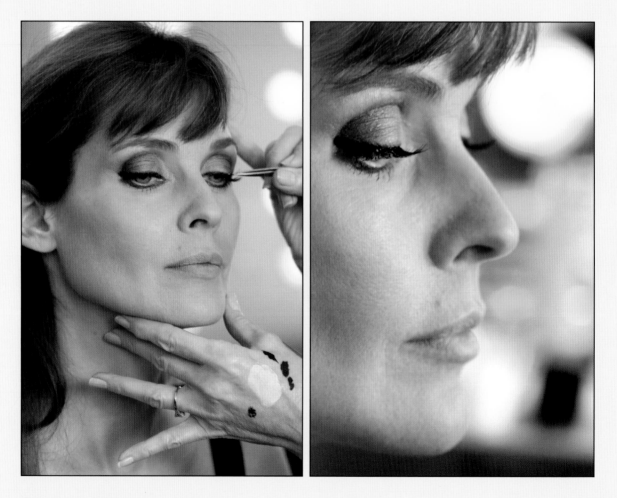

No-surgery Eye Makeup

Follow these makeup steps and you can't lose. They lift, sculpt, and dramatize your eyes. I use these tricks on all my clients, including Elizabeth Hurley, Cheryl Tiegs, Bette Midler, and Sigourney Weaver. You'll need about eight products, some good brushes, and a magnifying mirror. All the essentials are easy to find and available at every price that suits you, so check our shopping guide at the end of the chapter.

Take the extra five to ten minutes in the morning to do this eye makeup. It will give you an extra boost all day long and you won't need a touchup. To speed things up, keep all your essentials handy in a plastic baggie so you're not searching for them at the last minute.

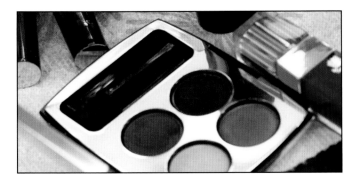

You'll need:

- **eye primer base**
- **densely pigmented black or dark brown eye pencil**
- **powder eyeliner or gel liner in a color complementary to the pencil**
- **soft crease pencil in taupe or brown (depending on your skin tone)**
- **crease shadow in a color complimentary to the crease pencil**
- **pale lid shadow**
- **eyelash curler**
- **black mascara**
- **eye makeup brushes**
- **felt-tip eye liner (optional)**

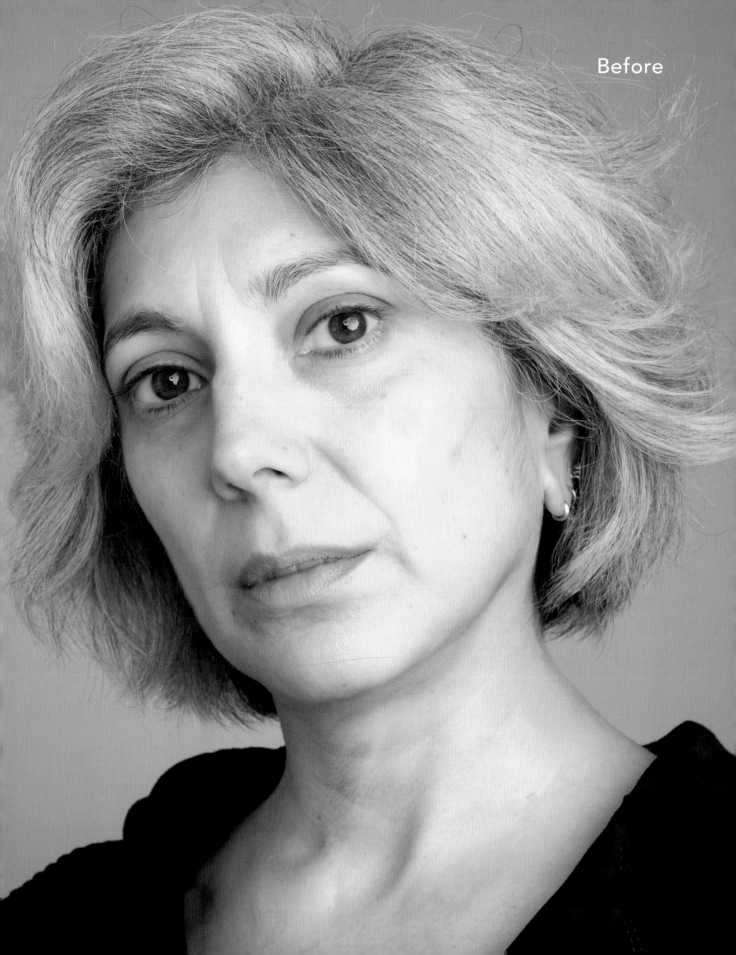

Before

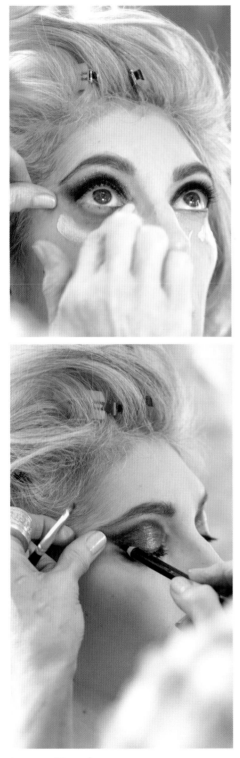

Lauren Ezersky

1

Do your eyes before any face makeup—even concealer. It's the pro way to go. This order surprises women because they usually do face makeup first and then their eyes. But during eye shadow application, shadow flakes always fall onto the under-eye and cheek area. Doing eyes first prevents double duty cleanup later and your foundation will look fresher.

2

Apply eye primer every time to prevent your eye makeup from feathering, creasing, and looking like an unmade bed. This is the real secret to great eye makeup. Primer needs to go on before anything else. It preps your lids from lash line to the hollow. Do you have hot lids or dry? Your answer will determine the kind of primer you need. If your eye makeup looks mushy a half hour after application, you've got what I call hot lids. In your case, a semi-matte primer like Laura Mercier Eye Basics or Lancôme Aquatique Waterproof Eyecolor Base will prevent your eye makeup from getting messy or disappearing entirely. These are tinted and can work as lid shadow too. If your liner skips as you apply it and powder shadows look chalky, you have dry lids. You need a creamier shadow base. You can also use a creamy concealer, like Lancôme Effacernes, or a nude color cream shadow as an eye base instead.

Dab your eye primer on the back of your hand first. Then apply it with your finger tip (not a brush) so you get a sense of the texture and don't overdo the application. A little goes a long way.

3 **Use a densely pigmented eye pencil in black or dark brown. This means the color is concentrated and opaque.** Not all black and dark brown pencils have high color density, so test liners on the back of your hand. Good liners will look solid on the first stroke and won't require work to build intensity. The pencil should glide on without smearing, but shouldn't be too dry or too

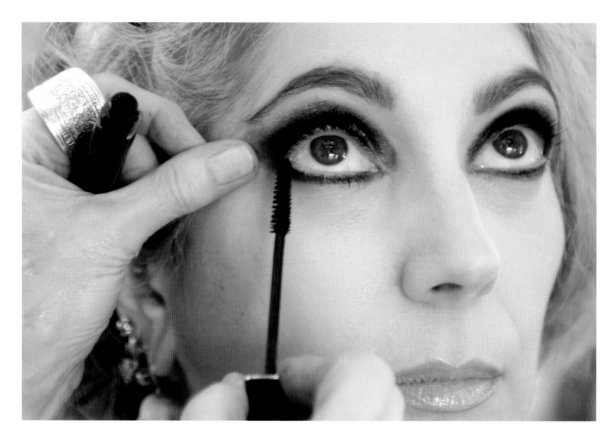

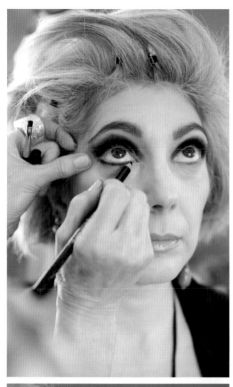

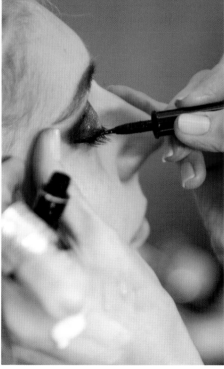

slippery either. Look for black pencils that won't go silvery, blue, or gray when applied. Master this eye lesson with black or dark brown pencil before getting into navy, plum, or burgundy. When you're adept at the technique and understand how critical depth of color is you can branch out.

4 **Gently pull your eye taut (but not tight!) at the outer edge to smooth the upper lid for lining.** This will help keep the line sleek and close to the lashes. Try to keep your eye open to control the application and prevent the line from getting too heavy. Keep your touch light. Let the pencil's density of color do all the work. Start sketching at the pupil and work outwards in slow dashes. Connect the dashes with a small, firm, and flat eye brush. Then go back a second time over your original line. This time work from the outer corner inwards. Thicken the line at the outer end now (about ¾ of the way out) to give the eyes a subtle lift; don't make the mistake of drawing the pencil up at the end in a wing though. Use a pointed Q-tip moistened with a dab of moisturizer to shave down mistakes like squiggles or where the line is too wide.

5

Kick the liner up at the outer corner with a pointed cotton swab. Moving the liner slightly upwards lifts the eye. This creates a wide-eyed look, counteracts sag, and draws attention away from darkness at the inner eye. Pointed swabs rather than the original round-tipped kind (which are too fuzzy and very annoying if fibers get in your eye) make a huge difference and are available at every drugstore. One of my private clients, a cosmetics guru, always says at this point in her makeup, "It's your happy eyes trick. You gave me those huge almond eyes again." Sometimes the smallest change makes the biggest difference.

6

Apply a matching "second liner" of dark shadow or gel liner directly over the pencil liner to build intensity. Choose a dark eye shadow or a gel liner that matches or complements the pencil liner you have just applied. For example, if you use a dark brown pencil, use a dark brown shadow liner. If you use a black pencil, use a black or charcoal shadow to re-line right over it. If you use powder shadow, make sure it's opaque and densely pigmented. Use a small, firm, flat eyeliner brush to apply the shadow or gel liner precisely over the pencil line. The shadow line will fuzz a tiny bit along the top edge when you do this but that's OK. It helps soften the line just enough without smudging it.

Gel liner applied over the pencil instead of powder gives a slightly different effect. While both shadow and gel intensify the pencil, gel gives a cleaner, sleek line, while shadow

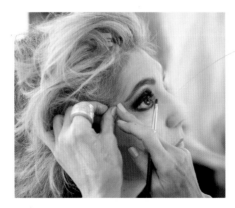

offers a soft smoky effect. Try shadow liner and gel to see which you prefer. Both add tremendous definition without a hard look. I always use pencil liner before lining the eye with powder or gel. The secret to fabulously lined eyes is drawing the shape with pencil and retracing with gel or powder shadow, or with liquid or cake liner. The pencil liner is the trick to shaping the eye.

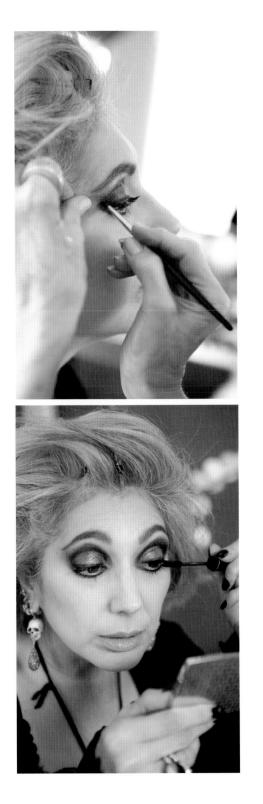

7 Lightly define the lower lid.

Use a light hand to line under the eye using a dense eye pencil—it could be the same one you used in step 6. Keep the top and bottom lines separate at the outer corner; usually, joining them drags your eye down in a Panda look instead of giving you the lift effect.

8 Contour the eye hollow to add depth and elongate your eyes—this is where the eyes get dramatic.

Apply a neutral, medium-toned pencil along the eye hollow right above the crease, just beneath the brow bone. Do this with dashes instead of a solid line. Blend the dashes with an eye brush. Women with light to medium skin tones can use taupe-y shades. Those with darker skin tones can use warm or dark browns. Usually, go lighter than your eyeliner for crease definition. Then retrace the contour with matching powder shadow. The pencil provides a base and shape for the powder to cling to, which is why powder shadow in the crease alone won't work. A small rounded dome brush makes tracing the hollow easy.

9

Apply a light-toned eye shadow over the lids for a clean, fresh look. It's the contrast of light lid, medium crease, and high-definition liner that make this eye makeup lesson work. This is why you cannot just do shadow and mascara and call it a day. Make your lids the lightest color in your eye makeup and never go darker than your crease color. Try shimmer because it can wake up tired eyes in an amazing way, especially in soft neutral colors like sand, apricot, peach, honey, or beige. Matte or satin shadows work too but stay away from heavy metallics. Being careful not to cover the eyeliner, brush on the lid color.

10

Splurge on a super quality lash curler and add black mascara that's compatible with your lashes. When it comes to buying lash curlers, this is not the time to scrimp on drugstore options. The Shu Uemura and Kevyn Aucoin curlers are worth every penny. Curl before applying mascara and use my maximum lift trick. Open the curler and place it as close to your lash roots as possible without pinching the lid. The curler should cup nothing but lashes. Turn your wrist upwards and away from you to get maximum curl. Slowly squeeze the curler closed for a few seconds and relax it, then pump again.

Use black mascara. Brown is my second choice. Select mascara according to your own lashes, not the final look you're after. For example if you have short, thin lashes, use a lightweight mascara to keep lashes separated and lifted once they're curled. If you have medium or long lashes with some natural thickness you're the right candidate for thickening, volumizing mascaras. If you're using a lash regrowth formula like Latisse you can use whatever mascara you want. Use mascara on top and bottom lashes unless your bottom lashes are very sparse. As you age, your lashes slowly get thinner. A lash-thickener formula might be too heavy. It can start to weigh your lashes down and they can begin to chip and flake during the day. Buy appropriate formula mascara for aging lashes.

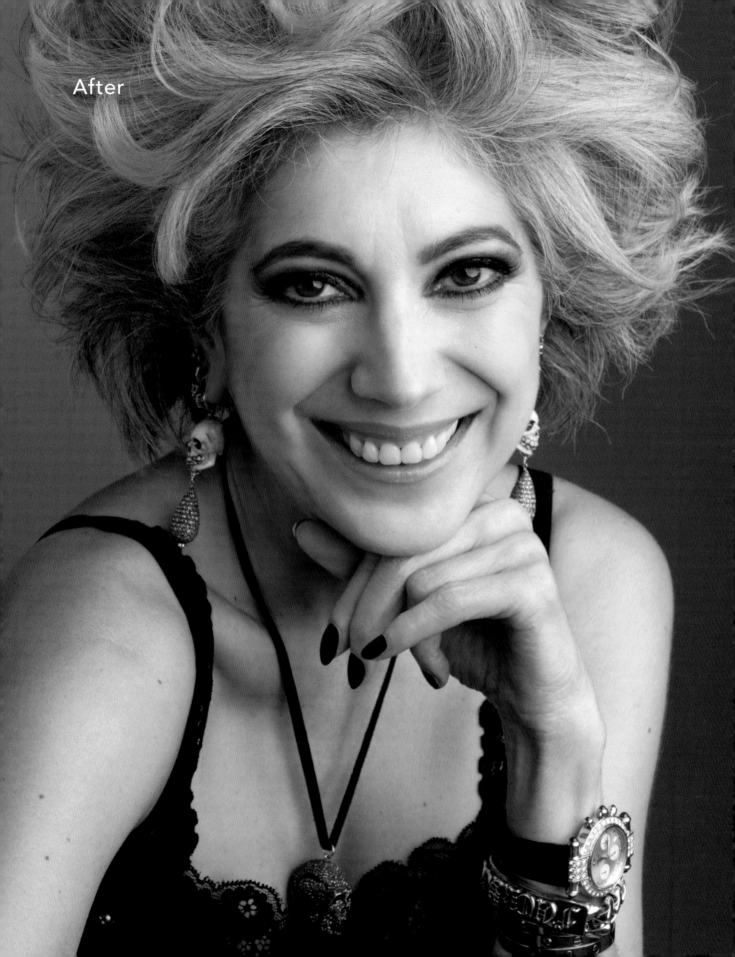

After

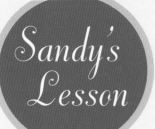

False Lashes

False lashes really add extra oomph to the eyes. Use dark lash glue instead of white for an immediate finished look (waiting for those white globs of glue to dry is such a turnoff). The dark adhesive melts instantly into your liner and your own lashes.

Choosing your lashes:

Individual lashes or flares come in tiny clumps of three or four lashes and provide the most natural look for upper lashes. This is definitely the best option if you don't want the lashes to be visible as fakes.

Full strips are wonderful for women who benefit from the extra line at the base of the strip. News anchors wear them often because of the eye accentuating boost they provide on camera. I have also noticed that these work especially well for women of darker skin tones. Check that the lash base is soft, flexible, and as thin as possible. Look for full strip lashes that are labeled "natural."

You'll need:

- individual lashes
- full strip, or flared sections that go on the outer eye
- Duo Eyelash Adhesive in Dark
- good tweezers like the Tweezerman Tweezer

Demi-lashes come in small half-strip sections and are applied to the outer half of the lids for extra drama. Flare lashes can be layered on top of demi-lashes for extra eye power in the evening. Once you become adept I think you'll want to wear them for day too.

Follow this routine for applying individual flares and adapt it for full strips or demis.

1. Use tweezers to pick up one individual clump of lashes right above the knot at the end.

2. Apply a tiny (and I do mean tiny!) dab of dark glue to the knot.

3. Holding the tweezers sideways and clenched shut, position the knot at the base of your lashes, right at the border gap where the root meets the lid.

4. Place the individual flares along the outer half of the eye, spacing them a little apart but not extending past the end of your own lashes.

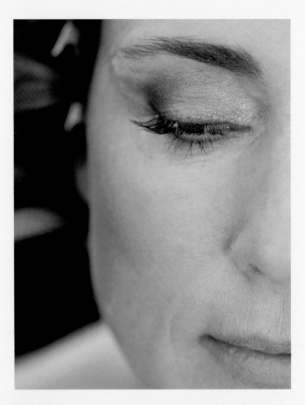

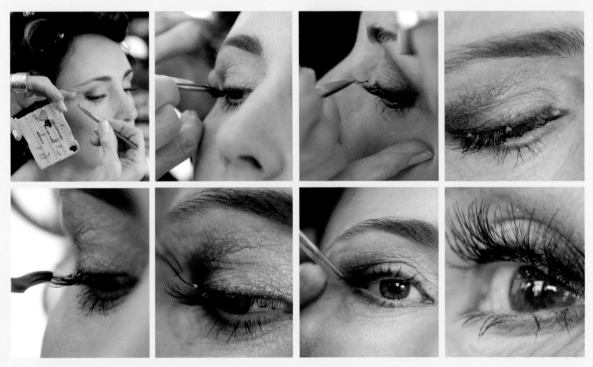

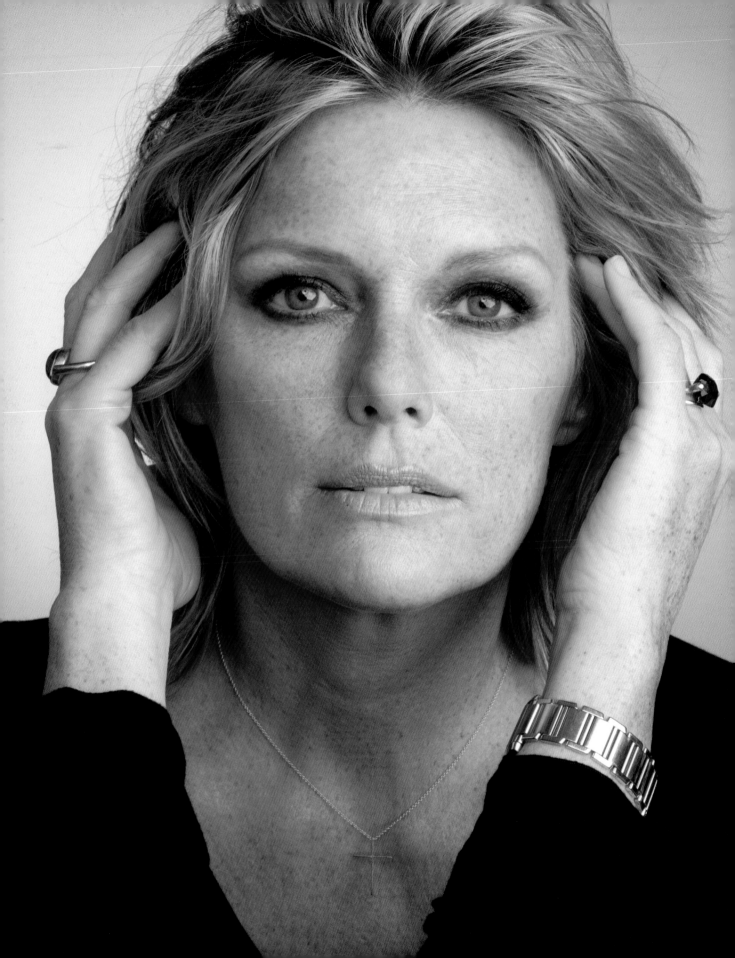

Patti Hansen

"Morning, noon, and night I love the look of smudgy, smoky eyes.

If you overdo it and your eyes look too hard all you have to do is soften them with a Q-tip; then go back at the lash line with a very sharp black liner to keep the intensity at the base of the lashes. I buy the Bobbi Brown Gel Eyeliner and her mini eye kits. I keep duplicates of them in my bag, bathroom, every- where. And I love false lashes. Everyone should wear them. I never used to do my brows but now, at fifty-four, I always do my arches—it gives my eyes a lift. Brows have become more important to my whole eye look than they were before. I don't wear foundation unless I'm going to be photographed some- where. The older you get the less foundation you need, I think. I love to outline my lips but the trick is not to see the lip liner at all, which makes choosing the right shade important. It should match your lips—mine is a beige-y pink color."

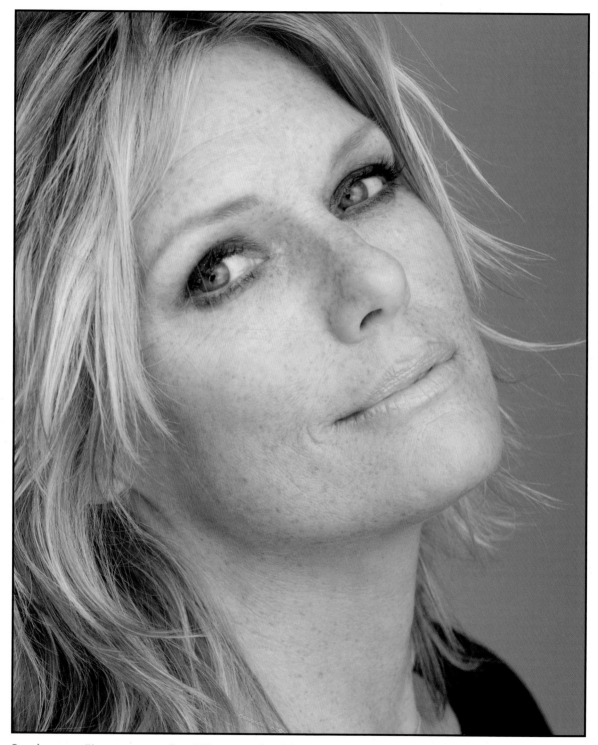

Sandy says, "I never want Patti Hansen's freckles to be covered; I just even out her skin tone."

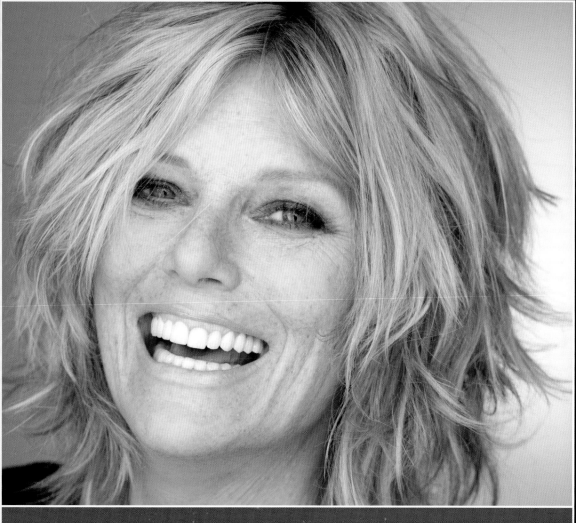

Sandy's extra special eye strengthening trick

This is a great tip for just about anyone but it's really effective on crepey lids or eyes with skimpy lashes. Apply a black felt-tip eye liner on the inner rim of the upper lid at the base of your lashes. To do this, hold the upper lid taut and dot the liner under the lashes. Connect the dots as you go to form a line. Don't use an eye pencil for this step—it will smear onto your lower lids! Felt-tip liner reinforces your eye shape without making you appear to be wearing a lot of makeup. The result is incredible definition.

I'm Obsessed with My...

Wrinkled eyelids: You'll do best with strong definition at the lash base. Avoid eye shadows. Emphasize eyes with pencil liner, powder or gel liner, curled lashes, mascara, false lashes, and Sandy's felt-tip liner trick (page 41).

Fine lines and crow's feet: Skip concealer and use a highlighter like YSL Touche Éclat at the inner eye. This will give you maximum benefits from doing your crease, liner, and false lashes.

Hidden lids: Don't try to contour. Dot a felt-tip liner along your upper lashes instead of pencil. Emphasize your eye shape with more defined pencil liner under the lower lashes and in the waterline (the lower inner rim).

Droopy lids: Blend your crease contour up slightly at the outer eye. Gradually thicken your liner on the upper lid and kick the line up. Highlight the brow bone with YSL Touche Éclat right below the arch.

Watery eyes: You're the perfect candidate for water-resistant mascara. Never attempt to line the inner lower rims or the inner corners of the upper eyes.

Red eyes: Get a bottle of Alcon Eye Drops. They're pricey but the best to combat this issue. Be sure to neutralize your lid color with primer before doing eye makeup if you have red lids.

eye makeup
secrets of celebs and models 40+

Celebs have makeup artists do their eye makeup. You'd be surprised how many stars get pro makeup jobs even for everyday neighborhood events like P.T.A. meetings or dinner and a movie with pals. Unfortunately, some get so dependent on this expensive habit. This is where you have an edge. Once you learn Sandy's tricks, you'll become your own expert.

They wear fake lashes. Models and celebs rely on individual lashes to supplement their mascara. They know the extra power of lashes shows up in photos.

Celebs tweak their makeup according to what, when, why, and where. They consider where they're going and what they are wearing. A simple black dress might require different makeup than a sequin-covered sheath or jeans and a jacket. Don't just apply makeup without a goal.

Models always have a pair of sunglasses at hand. They prevent squinting and protect eyes from the aging effects of UVA/UVB rays. This is a great suggestion for all.

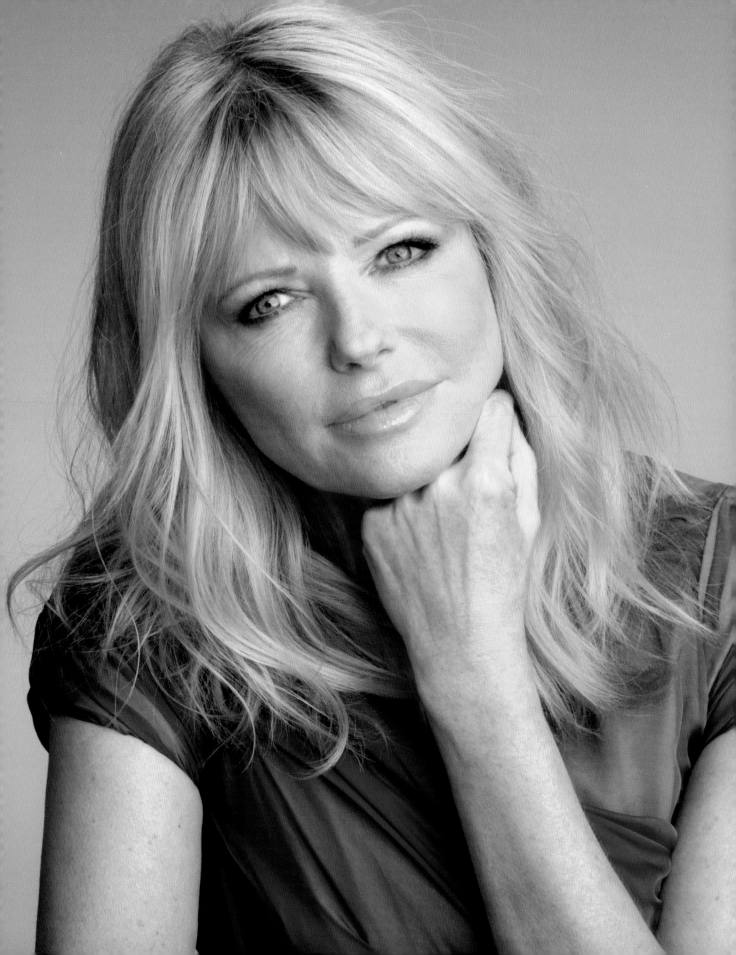

Cheryl Tiegs

"I took my looks for granted when I was younger, but all my life there were mornings when I'd wake up, look in the mirror, and think, 'Whoa, you need a little help.' As women get older they need to highlight the positive and be more selective about what they do. Someone once asked me how long it takes me to get ready for the Red Carpet. The answer is: a year. The way you present yourself is a cumulative package of drinking water, exercise, laughing, loving, and having joy in your life. It all shows on your face. At sixty-two, I know there is no magic potion. After all these years of having Sandy do my makeup—and it's probably around thirty years—I've learned a lot. There was a period of time when all I wanted was 'mermaid eyes,' sparkling blue and green and shimmery gold, for every shoot from sportswear to swimsuits. Sandy is always introducing me to new products. I also still get inspired by magazine photos and tear out images to copy the look. Doesn't everyone?"

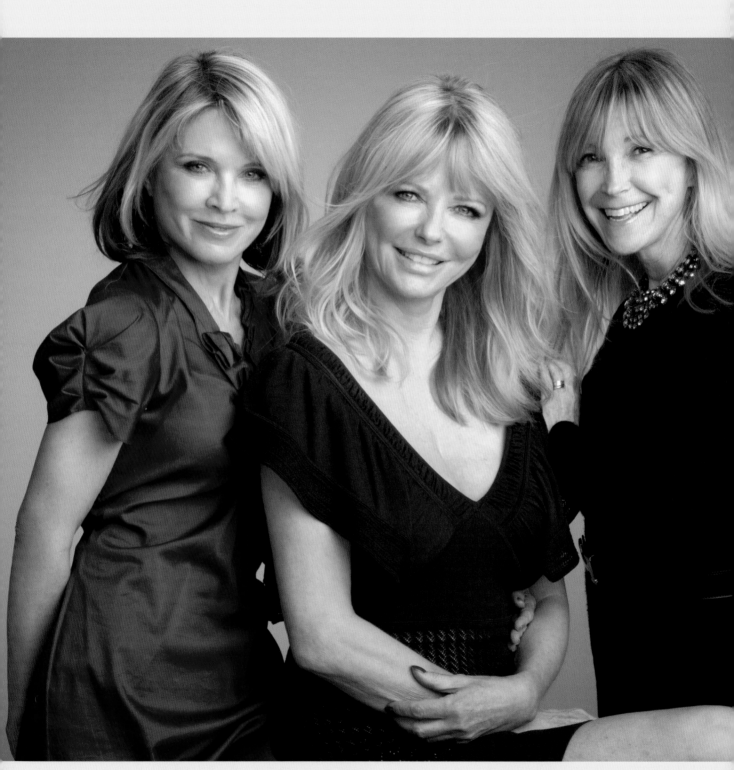

Sandy, Cheryl, and Lois, still working together, thirty years and counting.

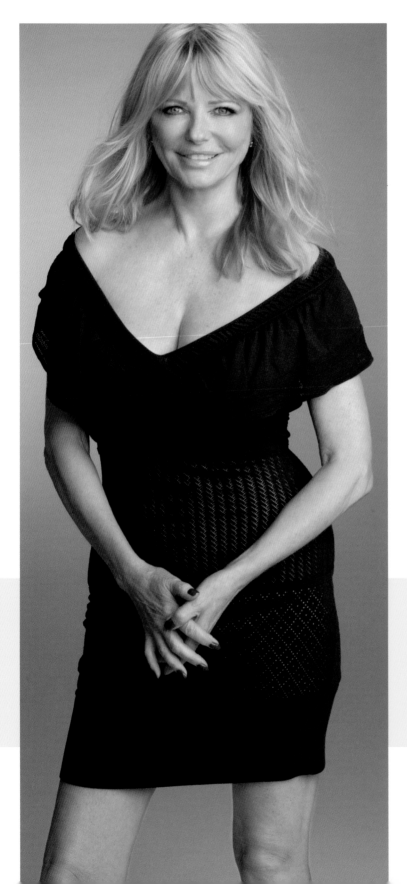

Sandy + Lois TIP

Stand back from the mirror and look at yourself full-length to get an idea of how your eye makeup registers from the distance most people will see you.

The Top Eye Makeup Mistakes Most Women Make

Hoarding. If your makeup drawer is filled with makeup mistakes and products from five years ago, toss them out. Now! You won't wear them. Besides, old eye makeup goes "off" in texture and color and can breed bacteria that cause eye irritation or infection. Mascaras and cake liners are the most vulnerable.

Serial shopping. If you've got twenty shadows by twenty brands and they're all medium matte brown or, all your eye makeup is one brand and has been for years, you're a makeup coward. What's the worst thing that can happen? We bet you always buy the same ice cream flavor too.

Avoiding aggressive beauty advisors at the counter. C'mon they're there to help and they might just show you something new. You will not end up looking overdone if you're specific about what you want. Say "I want to learn how to do an evening eye," or "My eyeliner is too flaky," or "I'm tired of matte taupe on my lids. What pale shimmers do you have?" Toughen up.

Using the applicators that come with the makeup you buy. Short foam applicators with stubby round tips make applying shadow difficult. Get a pro set of brushes and disposable pointed tip cotton swabs. You need a dome brush for the crease, one fluffy shadow brush for application, one shadow brush for blending, and a small, flat, firm eye brush for connecting pencil line dashes and applying a powder liner over pencil liner.

Neglecting to clean. We've seen

some pretty horrific makeup come spilling out of Hermès bags. Grimy, dirty makeup pouches with uncovered, dull pencils; sharpeners that have been used for eyes and lips; crumbly powder shadows; and mascara with grubby applicators. *Puh-leeeze* clean dirty brushes, sharpen dull pencils, scrape the top film off shadows that have gotten grimy, use wipes to de-grease and clean all your compacts, as well as the interior of the case itself when necessary.

Buying into trendy, of-the-minute colors. Those ads

of smiling twenty-something celebrities look cheery and compelling, but skip the bright blues, purples, and metallics. Once you get Sandy's eye lesson down you can play around a little more with color—one at a time. You might try a really dark, inky navy or forest green liner, or a shot of pale color on the lids like celadon, lavender, or amethyst while keeping the rest neutral.

Using loose or liquid shadow. Loose powder shadows just

make a mess. Liquid shadows don't blend. Skip them.

PROS+CONS

Like most friends we don't always agree and that's fine with us. My experience as a beauty editor and Sandy's as a makeup artist, in addition to our own personal preferences, mimic exactly what the women we work with say and think. Here's where we differ on eye makeup and why.

Q: **Eye liners. Automatic or sharpener required? Pencils or gels? Black or brown?**

Black can bring out eye color in an amazing way although women are sometimes afraid it will look harsh. If you've always used brown try a densely pigmented black pencil. Brown pencil gives a softer look but if you're going to use brown go for a dark brown or a black-brown shade. I prefer pencils that sharpen, rather than automatic roll-ups because I know exactly how much I have left. I hate running out unexpectedly!

I like waterproof automatic roll-up pencils because they're easier to control and they never require sharpening! I hate when my sharpener chews up a new pencil to a stub. Waterproof roll-ups are great for lining the lower rims if your eyes tend to eat up makeup quickly like mine do. Lately I like the look of gel liners too and have upgraded my usual black and browns to blackish shades of violet and green (Bobbi Brown's Long-Wear Gel Eyeliner in Black Plum Ink and Hunter Ink are my favorites). They give a dense lined look without a hard edge and are also smear-proof. Be sure to get a small firm eyeliner brush that's designed for gels.

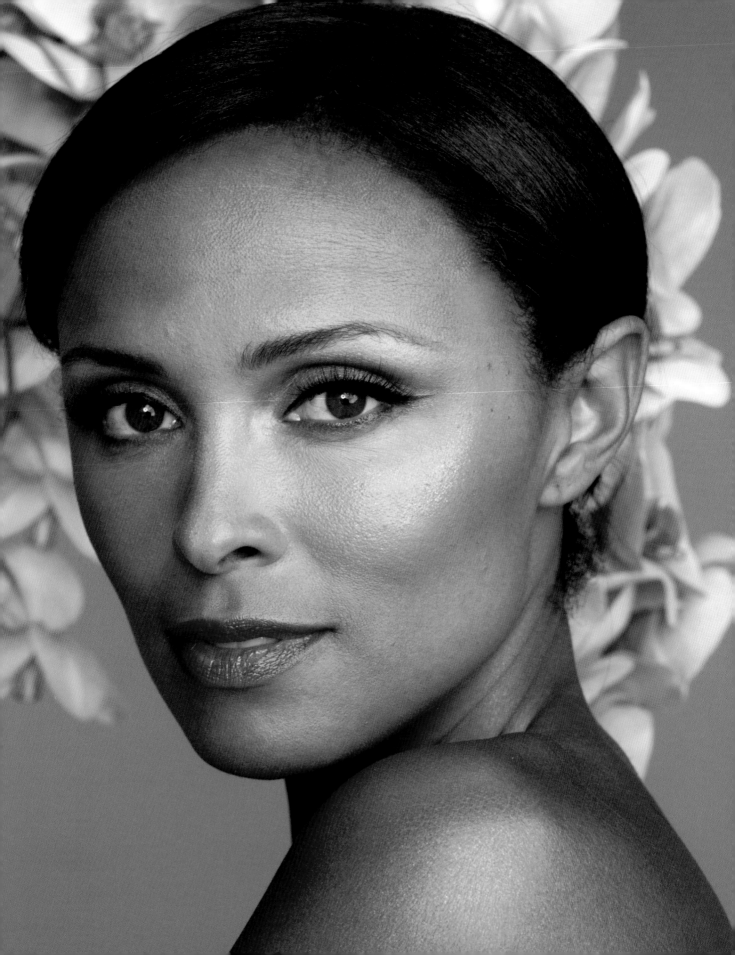

Q: Eye Shadows. Singles or palettes?

Mattes or shimmers?

Sandy says: Once again I look first for density of color. Forget about how a shadow looks in the compact. Test it on the back of your hand. You can't tell texture just by looking at color. Makeup brands designed by makeup artists are usually great as liners over pencil. They're very color and texture sensitive.

Lois says: I'm always hunting for eye shadow palettes with everything I need for lining, lids, and contouring the crease. Neutrals with a fresh spin—light to dark colors, mattes, and shimmers—appeal to me now more than basic earth tones of brown, beige, and gray. An updated mix of color and texture might, for example, be a palette with a shimmery peach for lids, a caramel color for the crease, a dark matte espresso for liner, and a sheer gold for layering.

Palettes are makeup simplifiers. They make travel and last minute makeup changes easy. Lancôme, Dior, and Yves Saint Laurent never fail to have amazing ones every season that are fully functional and provide most of your eye makeup. And by the way, NARS and M.A.C. make the densest shadows around.

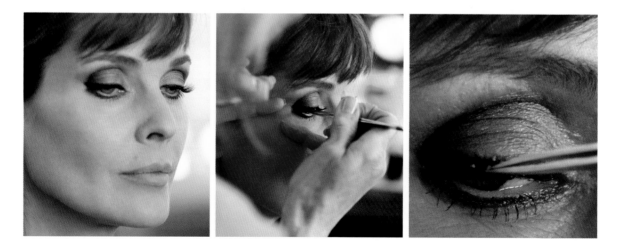

EXPERIENCE

- **Never apply pencils after eye shadow.** The one exception is cream shadow. Pencils can't glide over powder shadow.

- **Waterproof eye pencils develop a waxy film build-up.** This can prevent a smooth, dense effect. Make sure they're freshly sharpened before each use.

- **Let skin tone and eye color—not hair color—guide your choices.** Every redhead thinks she needs green eye shadow and every gray-haired woman goes for grays and it's just deadly.

- **Sometimes you just can't resist a trendy bold color.** Try incorporating the violets, blues, and greens as liners, not shadow.

- **You might go overboard on eyes and think they look too strong.** Brush a beige shimmer shadow or even a little loose powder on top to diffuse the color and take it down a notch.

- **There's a difference between smoky eyes and smudgy eyes.** Smoky is the one that works for us. Smudgy can look like a mistake.

- **Buy professional brushes.** They will last for years if you take care of them by using brush cleaner to maintain softness and shape.

Carol Alt

"My looks have changed and my round face has evolved into a more defined and sculpted look at forty-nine, which would have been ideal during my modeling days. Sandy used to contour my face to create the illusion of cheekbones that are now really there. **Today I do not leave home without mascara and lip gloss with matching liner.** My attitude towards beauty now is 'Whatever works for you'—if that's Botox or fillers, fine. On the other hand, I think nothing is more aging to a woman than a face that is too pulled back or too peeled.

I believe a raw diet de-ages you, but truly after thirty-four nothing is easy. I have my own Raw Essentials skin-care brand and I've written two books on my personal transition to a raw diet with lots of advice for women who want to make that lifestyle choice. There are lots of great recipes." (Check out Carol's products at rawessentials.com)

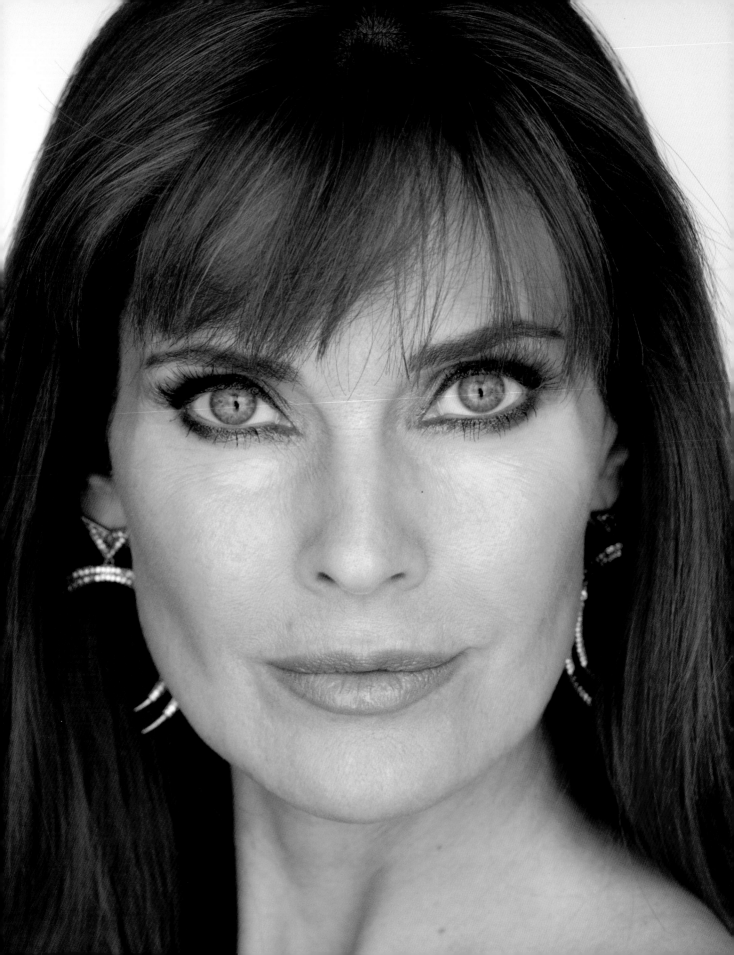

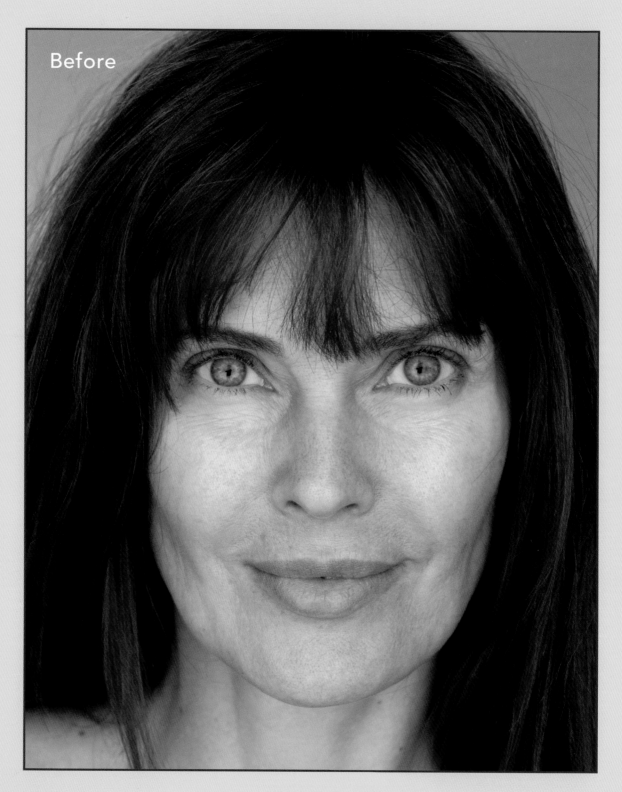

Before

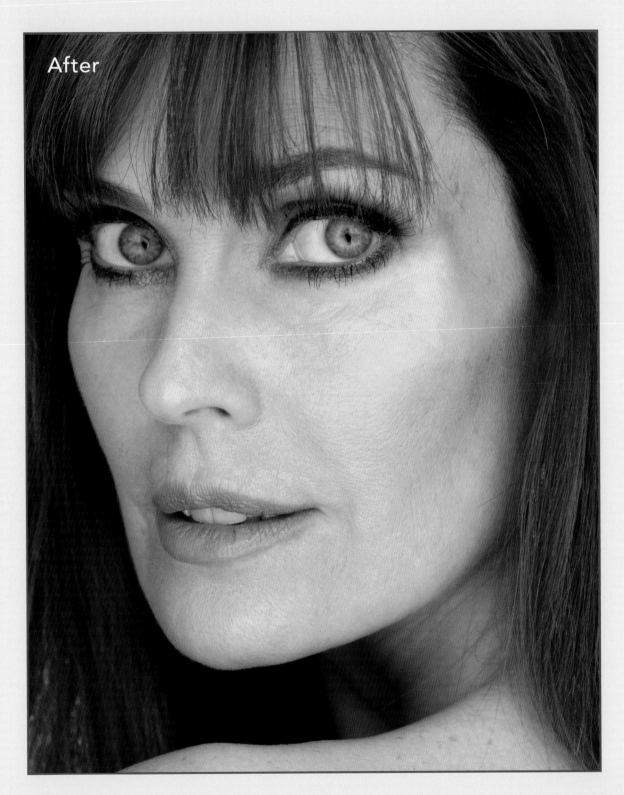

After

The beauty stalkers

Eye Primers

For hot lids:

- **Lancôme Aquatique Waterproof Eyecolor Base** ($24.50 lancome-usa.com)

- **Laura Mercier Eye Basics** ($24 sephora.com)

- **M.A.C. Paints** ($16.50 maccosmetics.com)

- **Trish McEvoy Eye Base Essentials** ($25 saksfifthavenue.com)

For dry lids:

- **Benefit Stay Don't Stray Eye Primer** ($24 sephora.com)

- **Lancôme Ombre Perfecteur Eye Shadow Base** ($23 lancome-usa.com)

- **Bobbi Brown Long-Wear Cream Shadow, in Bone, Sandy Gold, Malted**

  ($22 bobbibrowncosmetics.com)

- **Lancôme Effacernes Undereye Concealer** ($28.50 lancome-usa.com)

Eye Liners

Pencil liners with dense pigment in black or dark brown:

- **Chanel Le Crayon Stylo Yeux Precision Eye Definer, in Ebene, Espresso** ($28 chanel.com)

- **Giorgio Armani Smooth Silk Eye Pencil, in Black, Brown Black**

  ($27 giorgioarmanibeauty-usa.com)

- **Kevyn Aucoin The Eye Pencil Primatif, in Basic Black** ($24 kevynaucoin.com)

- **L'Oréal Paris Extra-Intense Liquid Pencil Eyeliner, in Black, Brown** ($8.49 drugstores)

- **Lancôme Le Crayon Kohl, in Black Coffee, Black Ebony** ($24.50 lancome-usa.com)

- **Laura Mercier Eye Pencil, in Black Extreme, Special Brown** ($19 lauramercier.com)

- **Maybelline New York Line Stylist Eyeliner, in Onyx, Espresso** ($6.95 drugstores)

go shopping for

- **NARS Eye Liner Pencil, in Black Moon** ($20 narscosmetics.com)
- **Shiseido Smoothing Eyeliner Pencil, in Black, Brown** ($20 nordstrom.com)
- **Yves Saint Laurent Dessin du Regard Eye Pencil, in Velvet Black, Leather Brown** ($28 yslbeautyus.com)

Dense powder shadows to layer as a second liner over black or dark brown pencil liner:

- **Bobbi Brown Eye Shadow, in Caviar, Charcoal, Smoke, Mink** ($20 bobbibrowncosmetics.com)
- **Giorgio Armani Maestro Eye Shadow, #33, #23, #35** ($29 giorgioarmanibeauty-usa.com)
- **Lancôme Color Design Sensational Effects Eye Shadow, in Guest List, Statuesque, The New Black, Backstage Pass** ($17 lancome-usa.com)
- **M.A.C. Eye Shadow, in Espresso, Carbon, Black Tied** ($14.50 maccosmetics.com)
- **Make Up For Ever Matte Eye Shadow, in Black 4** ($19 sephora.com)

Felt-tip and liquid marker liner for Sandy's strengthening eye trick:

- **Almay Liquid Eyeliner, in Black** ($7.49 drugstores)
- **Giorgio Armani Maestro Liquid Eyeliner, in Black** ($31 giorgioarmanibeauty-usa.com)
- **Lancôme Artliner Precision Point Eyeliner, in Noir** ($29 lancome-usa.com)

- L'Oréal Paris Lineur Intense Felt-Tip Liquid Eyeliner, in Black ($8.99 drugstores)

- M.A.C. Penultimate Eyeliner, in Black ($16.50 maccosmetics.com)

- Make Up For Ever Waterproof Eyeliner, in Black 1 ($22 sephora.com)

- NARS Eyeliner Stylo, in Nuits Blanches ($27 narscosmetics.com)

Gel liner as an alternative to pencil and shadow lining:

- Bobbi Brown Long-Wear Gel, in Caviar Ink, Black Ink, Espresso Ink

  ($21 bobbibrowncosmetics.com)

- M.A.C. Fluidline, in Blacktrack, Blitz & Glitz ($15 maccosmetics.com)

- Maybelline New York Eye Studio Lasting Drama Gel Eyeliner, in Blackest Black,

  Brown ($9.99 drugstores)

Crease Definers

Pencils for tracing the hollow of the eye:

- Giorgio Armani Smooth Silk Eye Pencil, in Gray, Chocolate Brown

  ($27 giorgioarmanibeauty-usa.com)

- L'Oréal Paris HIP Color Rich Cream Crayon Eyeliner, in Attentive, Meticulous ($10 drugstores)

- M.A.C. Shadestick, in Gentle Lentil, Taupographic ($16.50 maccosmetics.com)

- Make Up For Ever Aqua Eyes Pencil, in Light Brown, Light Taupe ($17 sephora.com)

- Sephora Jumbo Eye Pencil, in Beige ($6 sephora.com)

- Stila Convertible Eye Color, in Teak, Clove ($22 stilacosmetics.com)

- Lancôme Le Crayon Khol Eyeliner, in Gris Noir ($24.50 lancome-usa.com)

- Lancôme Le Stylo Waterproof Longlasting Eyeliner, in Bronze ($24.50 lancome-usa.com)

Shadows to layer directly over crease pencil:

- Giorgio Armani Maestro Eye Shadow, #20, #26, #28 ($29 giorgioarmanibeauty-usa.com)

- Lancôme Color Design Sensational Effects Eye Shadow Smooth Hold, in Mochaccino,

  Chic ($17 lancome-usa.com)

- M.A.C. Eye Shadow, in Cross Cultural, Wedge, Taupe ($14.50 maccosmetics.com)

- Make Up For Ever Eye Shadow, in Caffe Latte 164, Matte Beige Brown 163 ($19 sephora.com)

- NARS Single Eye Shadow, in Blondie, **Sophia** ($23 narscosmetics.com)
- Yves Saint Laurent Ombre Solo Lasting Radiance Eye Shadow, in Fawn ($30 yslbeautyus.com)

Lid Shadows

Shimmer shadows that make tired eyes sparkle:

- Bobbi Brown Shimmer Wash Eye Shadow, in Beige, Seashell, Champagne, Lilac

   ($20 bobbibrowncosmetics.com)

- Lancôme Color Design Sensational Effects Eye Shadow, in Gaze, Bikini Golden, Kitten

   Heel ($17 lancome-usa.com)

- NARS Single Eye Shadow, in Baby Girl, Fathom, Cairo, Edie, Nymphea

   ($23 narscosmetics.com)

- Stila Eye Shadow, in Kitten, Launey, Sun, Grace, Cloud ($20 stilacosmetics.com)

Matte and satin lid shadows that look clean and enhance every eye color:

- Clé de Peau Beauté Satin Eye Color, #103, #104, #105, #114 ($45 neimanmarcus.com)
- Giorgio Armani Maestro Eye Shadow, #1, #2, #3, #4 ($28 giorgioarmanibeauty-usa.com)
- M.A.C. Eye Shadow, in Shroom, Orb, Brule ($14.50 maccosmetics.com)
- Shiseido Makeup Luminizing Satin Eye Color, in Caramel BE202, Provence VI704,

   Lingerie BE701, Peach PK319 ($25 sephora.com)

Cream shadows for extremely dry lids:

- NARS Cream Eye Shadow, in Mousson, Corfu ($22 narscosmetics.com)
- Yves Saint Laurent Water Resistant Cream Eye Shadow, in Pink Sands, Amethyst Gray

   ($30 yslbeautyus.com)

Do-it-all Eye Palettes

For fast contour, lining, and shaping—multi-color palettes that really work:

- Chanel Quadra Eye Shadow, in Kaska Beige ($56 nordstrom.com)
- Clé de Peau Beauté Eye Color Quad, #2, #9 ($75 neimanmarcus.com)
- CoverGirl Eye Enhancers 4 Kit, in Coffee Shop, Urban Basics ($5.33 drugstores)

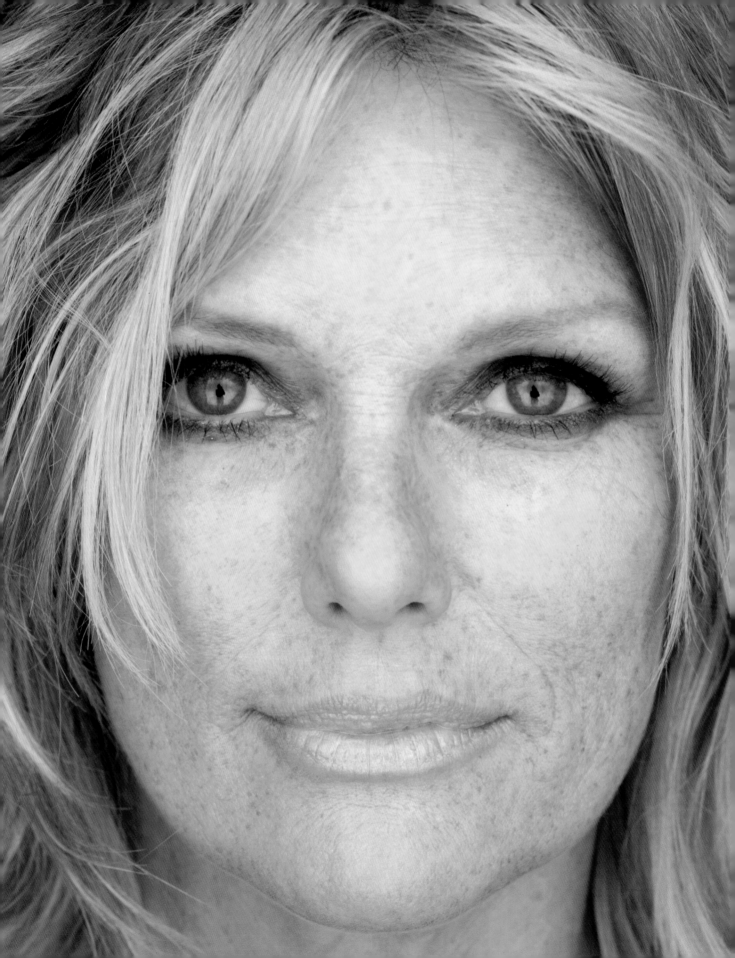

- Dior 5-Colour Eye Shadow, in Amber Design, Nude Pink Design ($58 sephora.com)

- Kevyn Aucoin The Essential Eye Shadow Palette, #1, #2, #3 ($55 kevynaucoin.com)

- Lancôme Color Design Sensational Effects Eye Shadow Quad, in Showstopper Style, Innocence Couture, Enchanted Evening, Glamour Era ($42 lancome-usa.com)

- Maybelline New York Expert Wear Eye Shadow Quad, in Chai Latte, Natural Smokes, Charcoal Smokes ($6.25 drugstores)

- Yves Saint Laurent 5-Colour Harmony for Eyes, in Sahara, Tawny, Bronze Gold ($56 yslbeautyus.com)

Black Mascara

Natural-look mascara for skimpy lashes:

- Lancôme Oscillation Powermascara ($34 lancome-usa.com)

- Chanel Inimitable Waterproof Mascara, in Noir ($30 chanel.com)

- CoverGirl LashBlast Length Water-Resistant Mascara, in Black ($8 drugstores)

- Lancôme Definicils High Definition Mascara, in Deep Black ($24.50 lancome-usa.com)

- Shu Uemura Mascara Basic, in Black ($27.50 shuuemura-usa.com)

Dense, thickening mascaras for natural lashes with body:

- DiorShow Black Out Mascara ($24 sephora.com)

- Estée Lauder MagnaScopic Maximum Volume Mascara ($21 esteelauder.com)

- Lancôme Hypnôse Drama Instant Full Body Mascara, in Excessive Black ($24.50 lancome-usa.com)

- Maybelline New York Lash Stiletto Voluptuous Mascara, in Very Black ($8.99 drugstores)

- Yves Saint Laurent Volume Effet Faux Cils Luxurious Mascara, in High Density Black ($30 yslbeautyus.com)

Eyelash Curlers

- Kevyn Aucoin Eyelash Curler ($19 sephora.com)

- Shu Uemura Eyelash Curler ($19 shuuemura-usa.com)

False Lashes

Individual lashes:

- **M.A.C. Lash, #30, #31, #32** ($14 maccosmetics.com)

- **Make Up For Ever Individual Lashes** ($15 sephora.com)

- **Shu Uemura Flare Lower Eyelashes**—use them for top lids! ($20 shuuemura-usa.com)

Full lash strip:

- **Laura Mercier Full Faux Lashes** ($18 sephora.com)

Demis:

- **Ardell DuraLash Naturals** ($3.99 drugstores)

- **Laura Mercier Corner Faux Lashes** ($18 sephora.com)

Eye Makeup Removers

For sensitive eyes:

- **Lancôme Bi-Facil Double Action Eye Makeup Remover** ($26 lancome-usa.com)

- **Lancôme Effacil Gentle Eye Makeup Remover** ($26 lancome-usa.com)

For desk, bag, car, travel:

- **M.A.C. Wipes** ($18 maccosmetics.com)

For removing lots of waterproof makeup easily:

- **Neutrogena Oil-Free Eye Makeup Remover** ($7.29 drugstores)

- **Yves Saint Laurent Eye Makeup Remover** ($30 yslbeautyus.com)

Eye Makeup Brushes

For connecting and blending pencil dashes, applying gel liner, or complementary shadow over liner:

- **Lancôme Angle Shadow Brush, #13** ($25.50 lancome-usa.com)

- **Giorgio Armani Eyeliner Brush** ($25 giorgioarmanibeauty-usa.com)

- **Kevyn Aucoin Eyeliner Brush** ($20 sephora.com)

- **NARS Push Eyeliner Brush** ($26 narscosmetics.com)

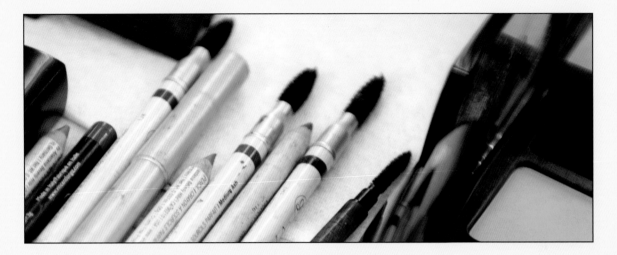

- **Shu Uemura Natural Brush, 5f** ($22 shuuemura-usa.com)

- **Yves Saint Laurent Eye Definer Brush** ($30 yslbeautyus.com)

- **Yves Saint Laurent Eye Shader Brush** ($30 yslbeautyus.com)

For doing crease shadow overlay:

- **NARS Small Domed Eye Brush** ($27 narscosmetics.com)

- **Giorgio Armani Round Eye Contour Brush** ($32 giorgioarmanibeauty-usa.com)

- **Lancôme Blending Tip Brush, #16** ($24 lancome-usa.com)

For applying shadow to lids or blending:

- **Giorgio Armani Eyeshader Brush** ($38 giorgioarmanibeauty-usa.com)

- **Kevyn Aucoin Medium Eye Shadow Brush** ($32 kevynaucoin.com)

- **Kevyn Aucoin Small Eye Shadow Brush Soft Round Tip** ($29 kevynaucoin.com)

- **Lancôme Blending Shadow Brush, #17** ($27.50 lancome-usa.com)

- **Lancôme Dual End Liner and Shadow Brush, #18** ($31.50 lancome-usa.com)

- **Laura Mercier Crème Eye Colour Brush** ($28 lauramercier.com)

- **Shu Uemura Synthetic Brush, #10** ($35 shuuemura-usa.com)

Brush Kits

- **Kevyn Aucoin Brush Set, The Mini** ($140 kevynaucoin.com)

- **Trish McEvoy Essential Brush Collection** ($150 trishmcevoy.com)

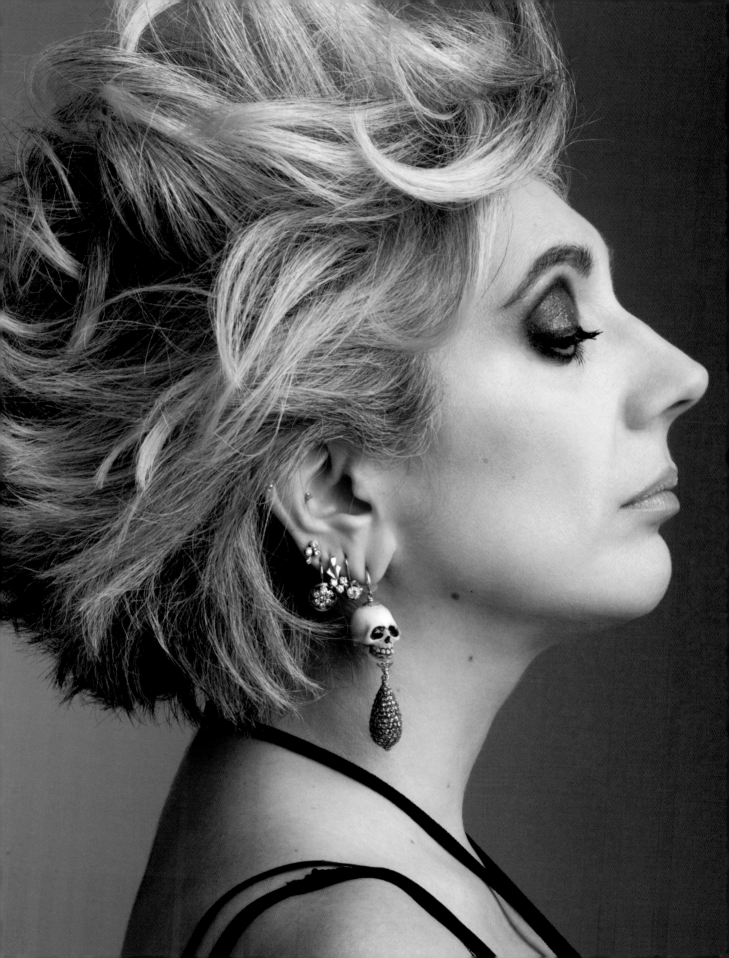

CHAPTER TWO

FULL, SHAPELY, MODERN BROWS

Brows are the shoulders of your face. They add definition, the appearance of bone structure, and attitude. Good brows divert attention away from crow's feet, dark circles, under-eye bags, and a saggy or plump jaw-line. Good brows are extended and full. Bad brows are too short, too skinny, or shaped like commas and tadpoles. No matter how cool and contemporary your clothes, no matter how great the rest of your makeup—if your brows are all wrong, you'll look out of date.

Please be cautious because we think at some point brows are all about filling in, not taking away. On women 40+ we rarely come across brows that can't use help. Here's why: during the '60s, many of us thinned, plucked, and bleached our brows to follow fashion. Unfortunately, in many cases they never grew back.

Laura Ezersky

The Better-Than-Before Brow

Every woman benefits from elongated brows that frame her eyes. We think brows should always be longer, straighter, and as close to your original, pre-plucked brows as possible. Once you get your brows back into shape all you need to do is maintain them. You want your brows to last forever—not be a trend-of-the-month item on your face. Certain celebrities, such as Brooke Shields, Elizabeth Hurley, Demi Moore, and Salma Hayek are known for their naturally strong, thick brows. Although they've modified their brows with age, the stretched-out shape remains intact. If you do the most fabulous eye makeup and leave your brows to fend for themselves, you've only done half the job.

Learn to shape better brows. If you've overdone tweezing in the past, makeup can help correct your mistakes and get your brows back on track. This chapter will make all the difference.

Your brows and eyes need to work together as partners. As a well-designed unit, they power up your looks and make the upper face a real focal point.

What was I thinking?
Or, My Life in Eyebrows
We've been there with you.

Every woman we know has brow horror stories of tweezing binges during her twenties and thirties. Fiddling with your brows when you're on the phone or in a mood is a dangerous distraction. Before you know it, you've plucked out way more than strays and stubble. Sandy and I both cut bangs at various points in our lives to let botched brows grow in. Some women just have naturally thin or weak brows. But sometimes a medical issue is behind brow loss at this age. Whatever the reason, make brow makeup your ally in improving bad brows.

You need to do three things: correct and stretch the overall shape; fill sparse areas; and control wiry, coarse hairs.

Brows are glam and there's a whole special niche of products to keep them that way. We have powder pencils, powder fillers, brow kits, tinted waxy gels, pomades, and marker pens in addition to the classic brow pencil. Brow enhancing is fun and easy for young women with their original brows, but we think problem brows for women 40+ is still a neglected topic.

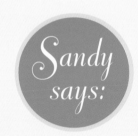

I followed the ins and outs of brow trends too. Fortunately, my brows grew back just enough so all they need is to be filled in with pencil. I need to strengthen the beginning, highlight the arch, and extend them slightly. This is my first year of coloring in the grey and I can do it with a pencil on its side, brushing up.

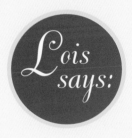

I've always had bad brows and brow envy. My own brows are weak, peak at the center, drop off halfway out, and have a wiry texture. I learned to love bangs early and made their camouflage my signature. But I didn't give up completely. Agreeing to try corrective brow makeup was a late-in-life lesson. Now on humid days I can finally pull my bangs back.

What the right brow can do for you now

Brows make a face look youthful and modern. They make you look polished and groomed too. Every set of brows is unique. Don't try to copy someone else's; although you can be inspired by a celebrity or model who looks something like you. Brows are as personal as your fingerprints. Getting your brows into better shape requires patience. The process is slow and similar to growing out a bad haircut—there are no overnight solutions. But it's possible to improve your brows in minutes with makeup.

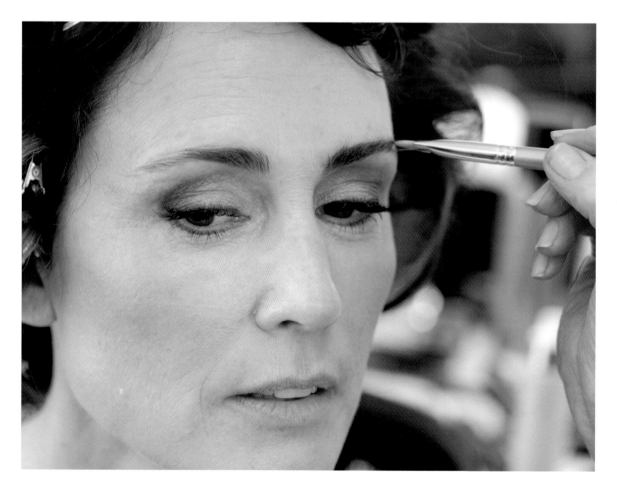

No-surgery Brow Makeup

My brow shaping and makeup lessons require discipline. Be prepared to let go of your old brow thinking. If you've never really worn brow makeup before your eye will need time to adjust to more definition. The success of your new brows depends on maintenance. You may need up to six products, but what you choose depends on your own brow needs. Here goes.

> ## You'll need:
>
> - **brow scissors**
> - **brow brush or spiral brush**
> - **brow pencil**
> - **brow gel or powder depending on your brows**
> - **angled brow brush (for gel or powder filler)**
> - **slant-tipped tweezers**

1 **Brush your brows up to see what you have.** Use a brow grooming brush with stiff bristles, or a spiral brush. This will make any gaps, bare areas, or poor proportions more visible.

2 **Trim long hairs with small scissors to refine the shape.** Leave the brows brushed up. Hold your forefinger horizontally along the top edge of your brows. Your finger acts as a guide and prevents you from cutting the brows too short and stubby. Snip the tips of hairs that are too long—that's the excess that remains along the top edge of your finger. Then, brush the brows down and carefully trim along the bottom

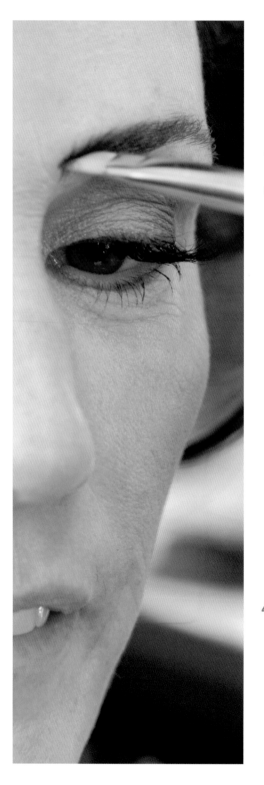

edge. (You can use this trim technique to groom your husband's brows too!) Caution: never use curved manicure scissors on brows!

3 **Choose your brow pencil shade.** Almost everyone can use a blonde or taupe brow pencil—except for the darkest brunettes. It's the shade I use on everyone from dirty blondes to highlighted brunettes. There are exceptions to a taupe pencil (and we'll get to those), but after a certain age you don't want a harsh brow. Blondes, especially pale blondes, should be careful not to wash out their brows by matching them to their hair color. You want the brow color to blend in with your own brow hairs. Blonde/taupe shades do that without overpowering your eyes. If you use powder or gel filler you still need pencil to create the basic shape.

4 **Define your arch and set boundaries for your brow shape.** The placement of the arch is the secret to a beautiful brow. The ideal arch is just past the outer edge of the pupil (not the center of the pupil). The brow starts on a diagonal from the inner eye and ends at a diagonal to the outer corner of the eye. The more elongated the distance between the beginning of the brow and the arch the better. Keep the outer half of the brow as horizontal as possible. Don't allow your brow to curve or angle down around the eye.

5 **Go back and sketch in the brow with your pencil.** Start at the inner corner near the nose. Holding the pencil on its side makes the pencil softer and easier to blend. Follow the brow shape in step 4 as closely as possible and softly fill in spaces to reinforce the basic brow line. Make sure the incline up to the arch is stretched.

6 **If your brows are sparse or missing sections, fill in with powder or gel.** A wax brow base will help powder brow filler adhere to your bare skin. These are sold separately and as sections in some brow kits. Take your angled brow brush, dip it into the brow powder, and lightly draw on the brow. Then skim the brush across the wax and go over the same area. This separates the hairs and helps the powder

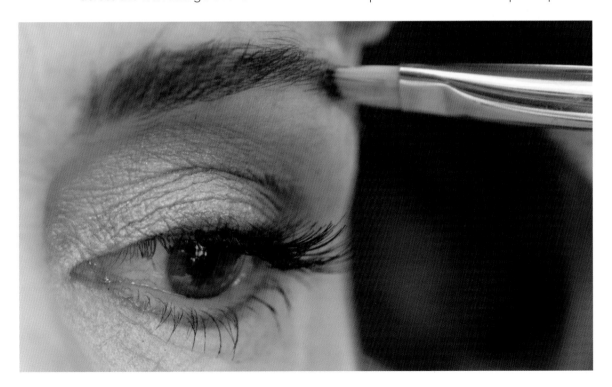

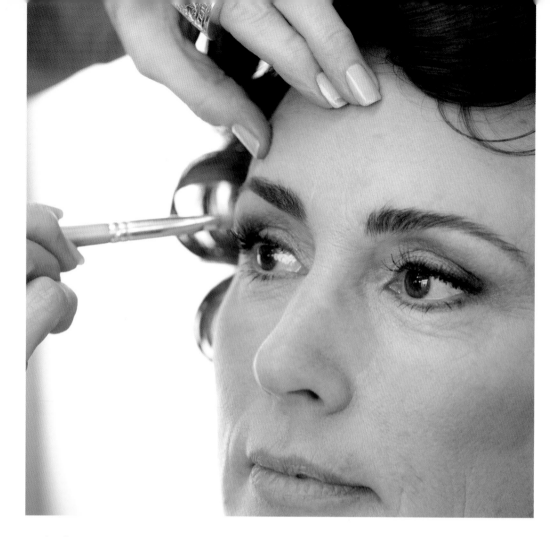

stick. If necessary, dip your brush into the powder again and repeat. You're essentially layering on color. A waxy gel like Laura Mercier's Brow Definer in Fair also works well and looks realistic when you recreate a missing brow tail. If your brows have the right shape and length but are not quite full enough, a powder pencil like Lancôme Le Crayon Poudre may be all you need. Powder pencils are dense and can be used alone.

7 Don't try to make your two brows exactly the same. The good brow always suffers. No two brows are ever exactly the same and that actually gives your face expression and personality. Don't aim for perfect symmetry when tweezing. Don't tweeze out gray hairs because they don't grow back and your brows will be left with permanent holes.

Julie Wolfe

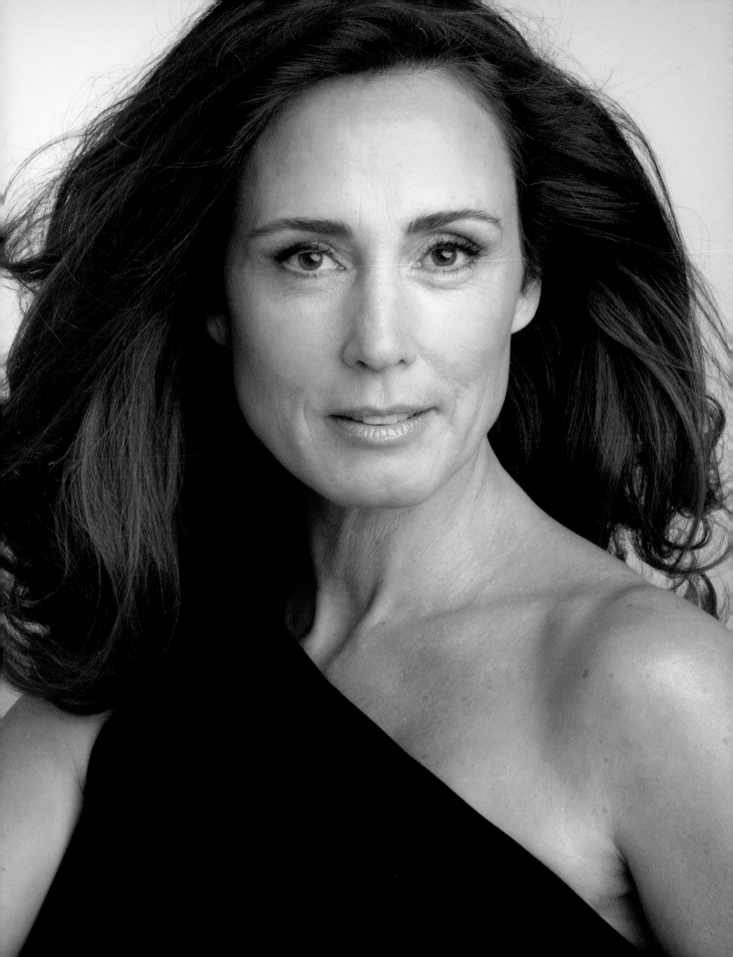

I'm Obsessed
with My...

Random wiry hairs: Control the extra spring and curl with brow wax or gel. A tinted gel is great for brows that are multi-color and multi-texture. Use it alone or over pencil.

Nearly bald brows: Working on naked skin is tricky. Use a powder pencil or the powder and wax trick in Sandy's brow lesson.

Tadpole brows: Growing out the shape may not even be an option at this point. Your goal now is to straighten out the shape with pencil and powder. Work on restoring a balanced thickness between the rounded starting point near the nose and the comma shape of the brow.

Saggy brows: You may have to tweeze or wax away the downward swoop of the brow entirely and recreate a more horizontal shape. Botox can help provide lift here too.

Botox brows: If you use Botox to help shape your brows, go to a dermatologist skilled in brow aesthetics, not just smoothing the forehead. Dr. Patricia Wexler says, "Bad Botox will give your brows an angry look or a clown-like expression by lifting the brows mid-pupil, into commas. Good Botox separates and extends the brow out horizontally."

Stubby, short brows: Stop trimming and tweezing for a month. Let your brows grow in and use powder or feathery pencil strokes to fill in the skin that shows between hairs for now.

Brows and eyeglass frames: Never try to adapt your brows to the frames! Reading glasses are often narrow in shape and brows show above the frames. Just do your brows and choose a classy frame that complements you. Black, taupe, or tortoise work for everyone, are never boring, and don't compete for attention with your eyes. It's time to resist anything cute, from leopard print frames to colors like red or tangerine. Be sure to choose frames that rest lightly on the bridge of your nose and don't leave an indentation.

Fake-looking dark brows: Sometimes all naturally dark brows need is a clear brow gel for grooming, no extra color. If you need a pencil for shaping and filling switch to a lighter brown or smoke color instead of black to take the edge off. Be sure to blend your brows and the pencil together to soften the effect even more.

Salt-and-pepper brows: Women with graying brows are usually ex-brunettes. Take your brows back to their original brown or smoky brown color in this case and skip blonde/taupes. You need the power of darker brows.

Brunettes who went red: Don't ask colorists to match your brows to your red hair. If you were a true deep brunette you're better off coloring brows an auburn or medium brown. If you have gone lighter red or strawberry blonde, an auburn or blonde pencil or powder can help make your brows and hair look in sync.

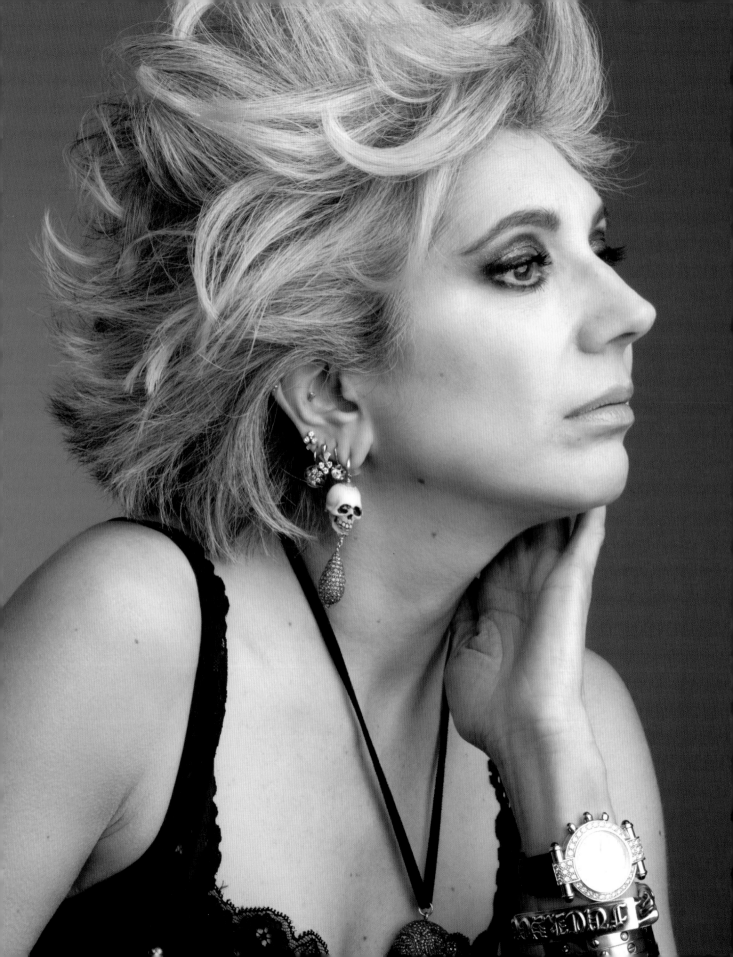

Lauren Ezersky

"I'm not the girl next door. I'm extreme about makeup and I feel naked without it. My eyes are my best feature so major brows and a heavy eye makeup is the first piece of my wardrobe. My brows are very strong naturally and I use makeup to keep the shape sharp and defined and cancel out the grays. My brows have gone salt and pepper now, at fifty-five, and I darken them back to their original color with makeup. Beauty is a fashion risk you've just gotta take. My hair started going gray in my thirties and I think it looks cool with my strong brows. I used to wear a lipstick for years that was very dark—the color of fresh liver. Now I wear a dark eye and a pale lip. The biggest mistake I see women my age making is they want to look the same in their fifties and sixties as they did in their twenties. I haven't felt the need yet for Botox or surgery but you never know."

brow

secrets of celebs and models 40+

Celebs make brow mistakes too. They just have makeup artists to get them back on track. When Sandy first met Elizabeth Hurley she had very thick Brooke Shields brows. "I cleaned them up just a bit but I was cautious. Elizabeth's father always said her brows were her best feature. Then during a mid-1990s fashion moment, a makeup pro plucked her brows to a skinny shape of two rows. Think back to Linda Evangelista and Madonna's brows during the '90s and you'll understand how drastic this was. Luckily, Elizabeth's brows grew back and have resumed best-feature status."

Models study themselves from side views too. The outer tail half of the brow is as important as the rest. It shows in profile. If you pull your hair back in a ponytail or wear it up in the evening, your profile is always on display.

Go to brow shaping pros regularly. Brow experts have become the norm at salons. For some women a brow specialist is part of their routine maintenance team. They schedule brow appointments along with bikini waxing and root touchups. And they make sure to give explicit directions so they stay in control of the results.

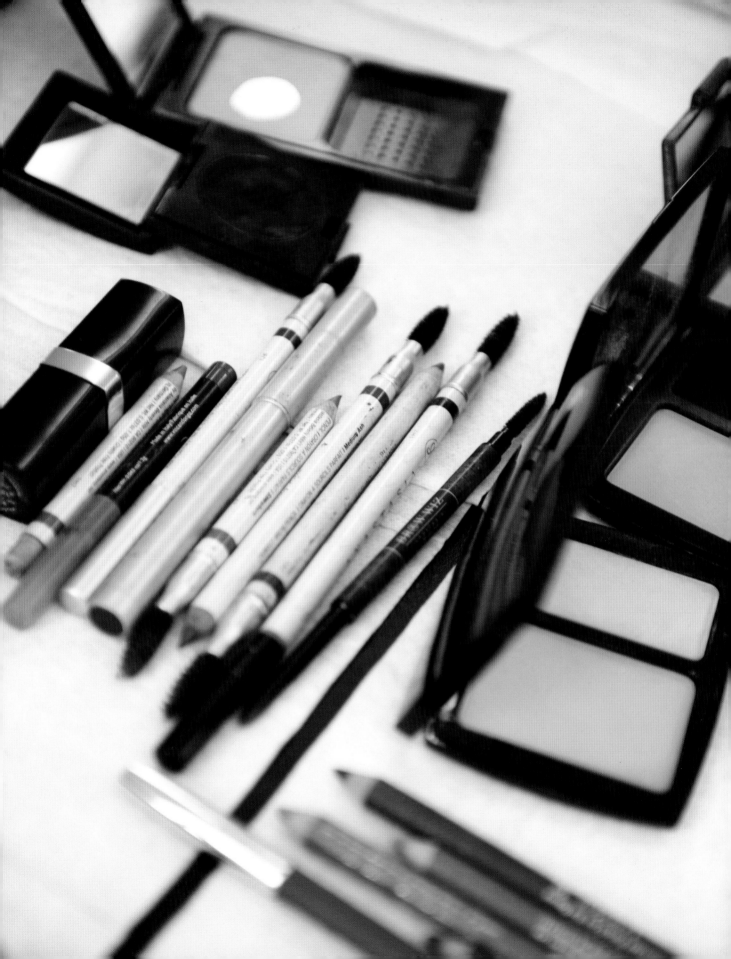

The Top Brow Mistakes Most Women Make

Going too natural. No matter how stylish you are, bushy natural brows need attention. You still need to brush, trim, and groom them.

Getting drawn into runway brow trends. Unless you're a very young fashionista who can carry off extremes, trends meant to exaggerate or eliminate the brows are not for you. We don't care if every designer and fashion layout has big Audrey Hepburn brows or Bowie brows bleached platinum—it's not age appropriate.

Thinking brow maintenance is too much trouble. Go to a brow pro who will keep them in shape for you. The payoff is worth it. Ask friends whose brows you admire for referrals, preferably a friend who trusts her brow groomer.

Not moisturizing the brow area. You need to treat the brow area as part of your face. Flaky, dry skin between and around the brow hairs inhibit application and looks like dandruff. Your brows need a conditioner. Use a balm to hydrate this area and double as a groomer. Be sure to rub your night cream through your brows before bed too.

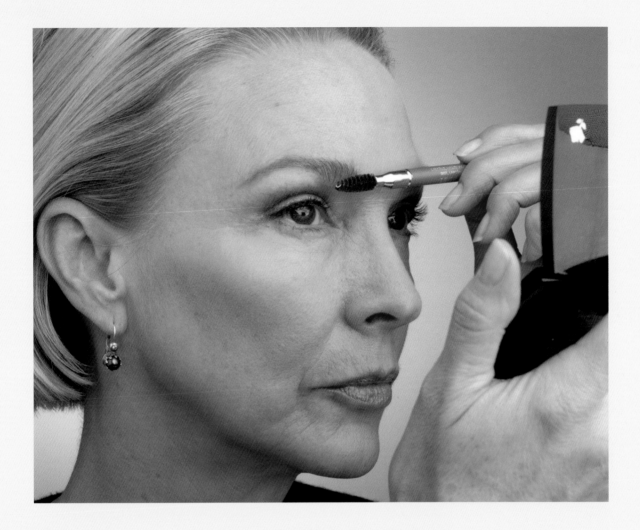

Relying on tiny tweezers and wedge brushes in brow kits. Brow grooming kits that include tools are great for travel but not for everyday care. Use the powder and wax but get good full-sized tools.

Extremely peaked brows. Sharp arched brows with a high peak give your face an angry or haughty look. Try to reshape them for a softer line with a lower arch.

PROS+CONS

We totally agree that brows can make or break your looks. However, our own personal and professional experiences have shaped our brow makeup opinions. Sandy has good enough brows and I have difficult ones. Here's where we differ and why.

Q: • **Brow pencil.**
• **Color and texture?**

For starters, never use eyeliner pencil to double as a brow pencil because it is too soft and will smear. I prefer using brow pencils to any other brow makeup whenever possible. They are usually hard in texture so they do not transfer, bleed, or smear. If your brows are basically good and you've been maintaining them, a pencil and a brow brush are all you need. Blondes and highlighted brunettes should stick with taupe or blonde, true brunettes should soften up to brown, and gray-haired women should go back to their original shade.

Taupe/blonde pencils are fantastic for women like me, who are tentative about brow makeup but need lots of daily filling and reshaping. They help you correct without being obvious and are practically foolproof. Tweezing away my droopy outer brow and sketching in a new one is now my favorite trick. Keep an open mind. It is possible to change a brow you've felt stuck with for years.

Brow powder or

wax-gel fillers?

I like both. I suggest the wax-gels or a powder pencil to clients who need to recreate the beginning or outer half of their brows from scratch. It requires some skill, but a spiral brush can soften the gel or powder application. Always brush through brows after any brow product.

I love the new wax-gels for their staying power, but for random beefing up, powder pencils are fast. I keep one in my bag for retouches.

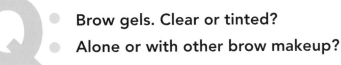

Brow gels. Clear or tinted?

Alone or with other brow makeup?

I think brow gels in mascara-like wands are essential for keeping wiry, coarse brow hairs flat and in line. Gels can be used as a final grooming step over pencils. Some gels come in color and can be used alone instead of pencil or powder.

Tinted gels train brows while adding a subtle fullness. Think of how a gel styling product works for your hair. Brow gel keeps curly, springy hairs in place and are great for weekends and casual days when you just don't feel like doing full makeup on your brows.

Karen Bjornson

"I started modeling in 1970. A month after arriving in New York I was lucky enough to be introduced to the designer Halston, who was looking for a new house model. Halston was an educator. In those days we did our own hair and makeup for shoots and runway so I learned what works for me. My motto at fifty-eight is, 'This is as good as it gets today.' Looking good at any age is about maintenance. When my teeth started shifting a few years ago, I used Invisalign and I've had Botox for the frown line between my brows. I think the biggest mistake women my age make is going to extremes— either they do too much or not enough."

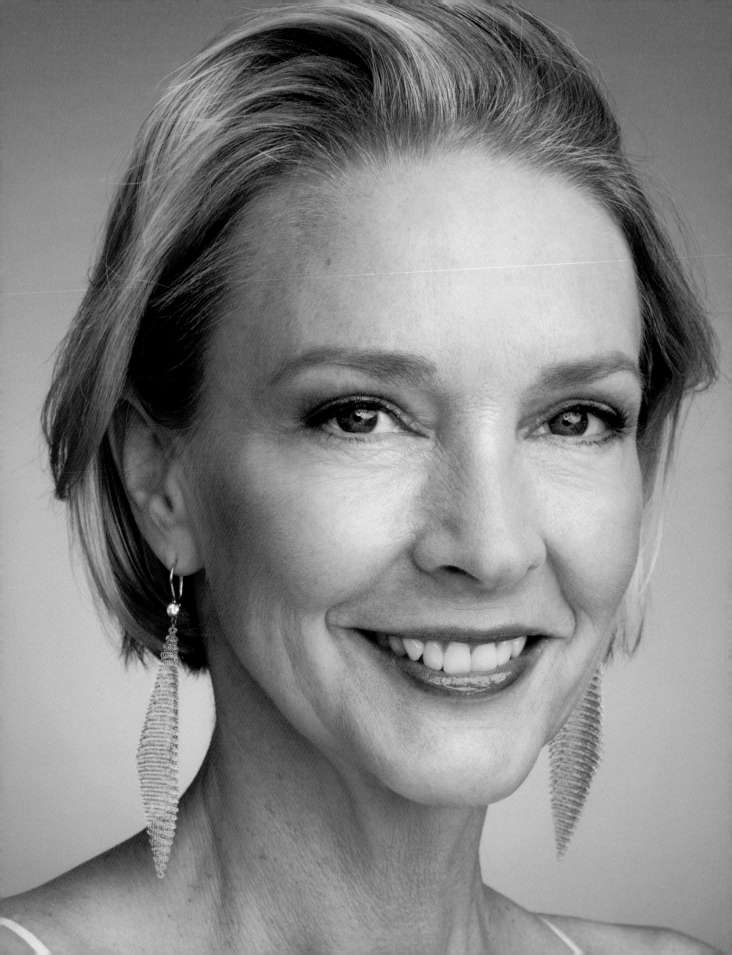

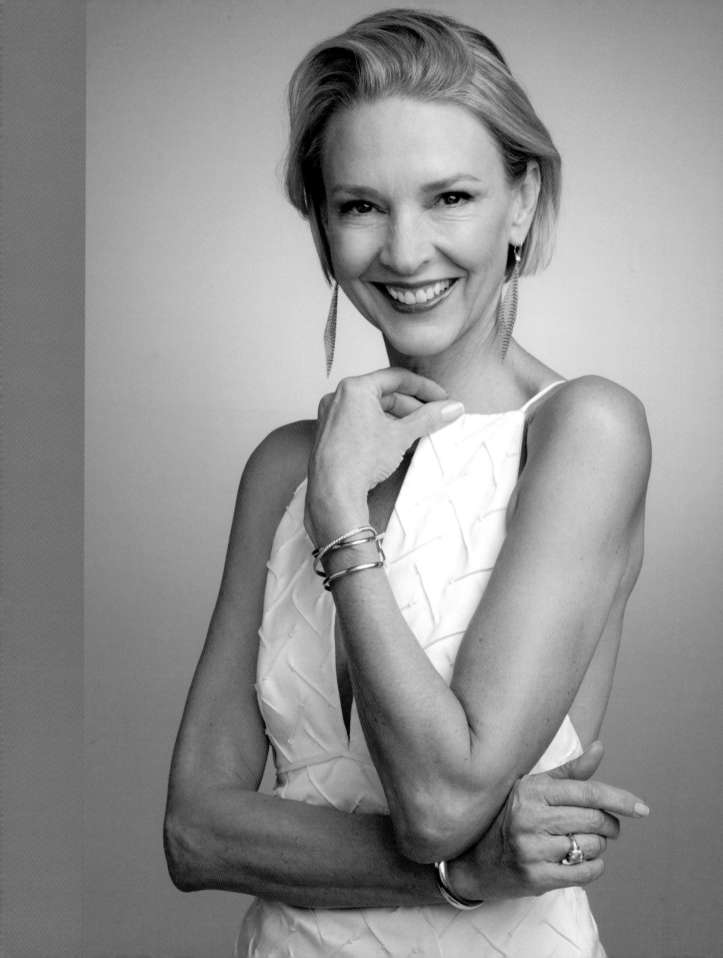

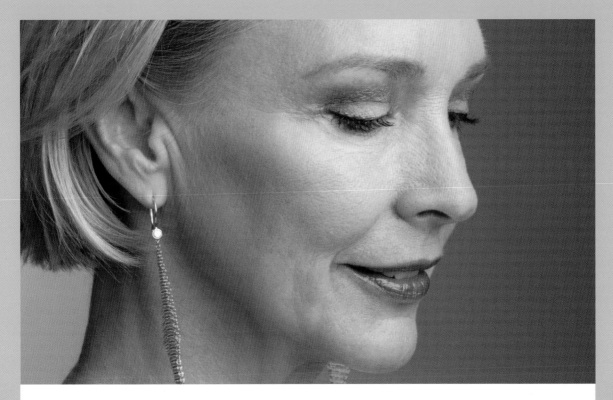

EXPERIENCE

C O U N T S

- **Fill in very sparse, bare areas first.** You want to avoid adding too much color where it's not needed. This is especially true with powder brow makeup, which is more pigmented and dense.

- **If you splurge on one brow product, make it a good tweezer.** The pricier ones are refined at the tip, won't pinch, and have more spring so you have more control. Save the plastic nub that protects the tip.

The beauty stalkers

Brow pencils

Taupe and blonde pencils that work for almost everyone:

- **Anastasia Beverly Hills Perfect Brow Pencil, in Ash Blonde, Taupe, Blonde** ($22 anastasia.net)
- **Bobbi Brown Brow Pencil, in Blonde, Wheat** ($20 bobbibrowncosmetics.com)
- **Kevyn Aucoin The Precision Brow Pencil, in Blonde** ($24 kevynaucoin.com)
- **L'Oréal Custom Brow Shaping Pencil, in Blonde** ($8.99 drugstores)
- **M.A.C. Impeccable Brow Pencil, in Blonde, Dirty Blonde, Taupe** ($15 maccosmetics.com)
- **Maybelline Define-a-Brow Eyebrow Pencil, in Dark Blonde, Light Blonde** ($6.95 drugstores)

Dark brown or smoke pencils for gray/salt-and-pepper brows:

- **Bobbi Brown Brow Pencil, in Mahogany, Ash** ($20 bobbibrowncosmetics.com)
- **Chanel Le Crayon Sourcils Precision Brow Definer, in Soft Brown, Cendre Noir** ($28 chanel.com)
- **Laura Mercier Eyebrow Pencil, in Brunette, Warm Brunette** ($19 sephora.com)

For redheads/auburn brownettes:

- **Anastasia Beverly Hills Perfect Brow Pencil, in Strawburn** ($22 anastasia.net)
- **Kevyn Aucoin The Precision Brow Pencil, in Auburn** ($24 kevynaucoin.com)

Powder pencils

For filling and extending skimpy brows:

- **Dior Powder Eyebrow Pencil, in Blonde, Brown, Chestnut, Sable** ($28 neimanmarcus.com)
- **Lancôme Le Crayon Poudre Powder Pencil for Brows, in Natural Blonde, Brunet, Taupe, Sable, Chataigne** ($24 lancome-usa.com)
- **L'Oréal Paris Brow Stylist Professional Brow, in Blonde** ($9.95 drugstores)

go shopping for

Waterproof brow gel + cream fillers

For very bare, balding, misshaped brows or brows missing a tail:

- **Laura Mercier Brow Definer, in Fair, Soft, Warm** ($20 sephora.com)
- **Make Up For Ever Waterproof Eyebrow Corrector, #0, #2, #3**

  ($19 sephora.com)

Brow powder duos

- **Anastasia Brow Powder Duo, in Ash Blonde, Golden Blonde, Strawburn, Medium Ash, Brunette** ($22 anastasia.net)
- **Laura Mercier Brow Powder Duo, in Deep Blonde, Brunette, Auburn, Ash** ($24 lauramercier.com)

Wax + powder filler kits

- **Clarins Pro Palette Eyebrow Kit** ($35 us.clarins.com)
- **Smashbox Brow Tech, in Blonde, Taupe, Auburn, Soft Brown, Brunette** ($24 sephora.com)
- **Anastasia Brows, in Bloom** ($28 anastasia.net)

Gel wands

Tinted gel groomer for coloring and controlling wiry, curly, coarse, or difficult brows:

- **Anastasia Beverly Hills Tinted Brow Gel, in Blonde, Caramel,**

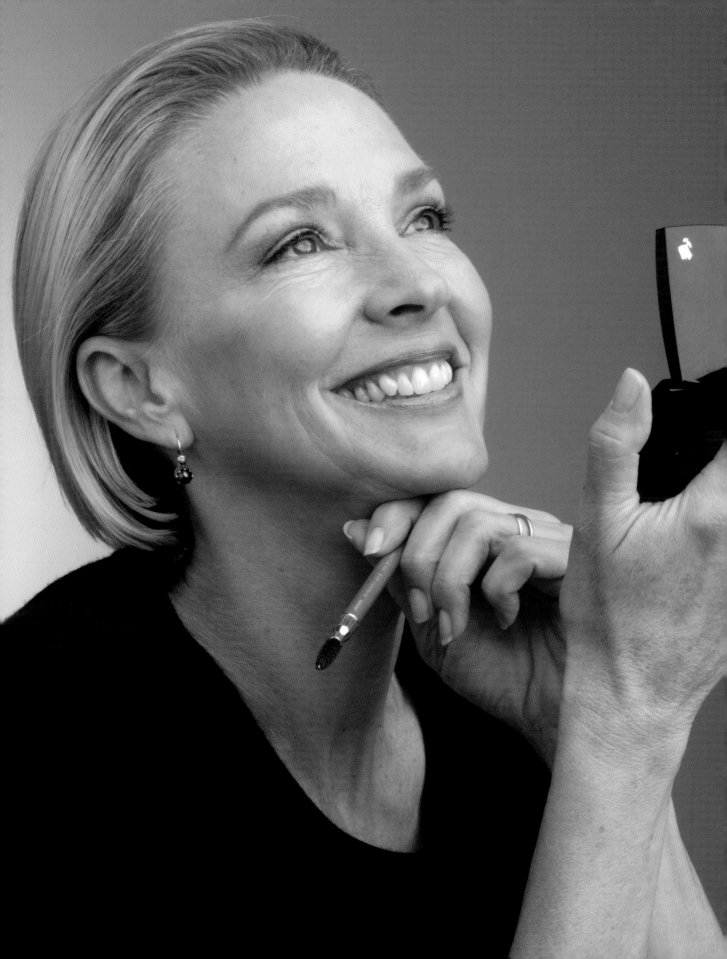

Brunette, Espresso, Granite ($21 anastasia.net)

- **Dior DiorShow Tinted Brow Gel, in Shiny Blond, Shiny Brown** ($17.50 sephora.com)
- **Lancôme Modele Sourcils Brow Groomer, in Taupe, Brunet** ($22 lancome-usa.com)
- **M.A.C. Brow Set, in Girl Boy, Beguile, Show-Off** ($15 maccosmetics.com)

Clear groomers

Mascara-like wands of transparent gel:

- **Ardell Sculpting Gel** ($4.09 drugstores)
- **Giorgio Armani Eyebrow Defining Gel** ($26 giorgioarmanibeauty-usa.com)
- **Lancôme Modele Sourcils Brow Groomer, in Naturel** ($22 lancome-usa.com)
- **Revlon Brow Styling Gel** ($5.99 drugstores)

Brow wax

To hold powder in place:

- **Anastasia Beverly Hills Brow Fix** ($21 anastasia.net)
- **M.A.C. Brow Finisher** ($15 maccosmetics.com)

Tools

Brow scissors for trimming long brow hairs:

- **Anastasia Beverly Hills Brow Scissors** ($22.50 anastasia.net)
- **CoverGirl Brow Grooming Kit** ($10 drugstores)

Tweezers for shaping brows:

- **Tweezerman Slant Tweezer** ($20 tweezerman.com)

Brow brushes for applying powder, gel, or cream fillers:

- **Laura Mercier Brow Definer Brush** ($20 lauramercier.com)
- **Make Up For Ever Eyebrow Brush** ($19 sephora.com)
- **Smashbox Angle Brow Brush, #12** ($19 smashbox.com)

CHAPTER THREE

A Smoother, Fresher Face

A great foundation is the make-up equivalent of the perfect bra.

Nothing beats it for boosting your confidence and keeping secrets undercover. Unfortunately, finding the perfect foundation is difficult and the confusion is due in part to the claims made on the label. Foundations that claim to firm your skin and provide an airbrushed look are not miracles in a jar. Foundation, or "base" as we sometimes call it, continues to be the most frustrating makeup item of all to buy and wear.

Alva Chinn

The Grown-up Face

If you wear foundation and use the right color, texture, and technique, you ARE going to look younger than if you don't wear makeup.

Here's the truth: Women do get wrinkles and makeup doesn't cover them. Many women forgo foundation because they think it emphasizes wrinkles and makes them look old. It certainly can if you choose the wrong one and apply it incorrectly! But by giving up on foundation you're cheating your face out of its best look.

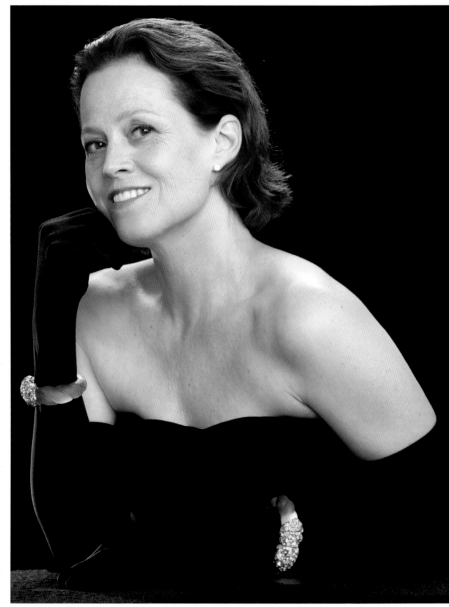

Sigourney Weaver

What was I thinking?
Or, My Life in Foundation
We've been there with you.

You cannot skip foundation anymore. Facing the day bare faced at fifty is a lot different than it was at twenty-five or even thirty-five. Young women look fabulous straight out of the shower, in wet hair and flip-flops with no makeup. At fifty you want a little more help but you don't want to look overdone either. Makeup brands are taking our dilemma seriously and keep bumping up the category of foundations that target our demo every season. Foundations now boast about their firming, lifting, tightening, smoothing, nourishing, and radiance-boosting capabilities. The ingredient lists sound a lot like those for wrinkle creams. Practically every foundation is packed with antioxidants, vitamins, collagen, peptides, botanicals, minerals, and sunscreen. Who doesn't want to look more luminous and get extra de-aging benefits just by putting on makeup every day? We're not against anti-aging foundations but . . .

Here's the catch—women get too caught up in the "anti-aging" part and forget that when it comes to selecting foundation it's really all about color and texture.

Even if you have a facelift, you still need foundation. Surgery can tighten saggy tissue and give you a crisp jaw line, but it doesn't change skin texture and pigmentation problems on the surface. Only laser resurfacing or a peel can change that and even then you still need foundation.

Right now you're probably settling with one or two choices and are not truly happy. You need a better foundation or a smarter technique for application and that's where we come in. Keep reading. We've done the legwork, or rather the facework, for you and we have the answers you need.

Sandy says: I've worn full-face makeup every day of my life since the '60s—even to the beach. Foundation had no SPF back then but it was still a great barrier against the sun. This was way before the idea of sun protection existed. To this day I believe makeup helped save my skin. When I was young, concealer was much more important to me than foundation. And now it is the reverse, the reason being that as you age, the skin gets thinner and concealer is too heavy. The foundation just has to work harder for you. I never choose makeup for its anti-aging benefits. I choose moisturizer for that purpose. I love foundation for its instant gratification. I try new formulas and update my own personal makeup and my professional kit constantly. I get tremendous feedback from my huge variety of real-life clients. I do test makeup on clients. There isn't any other way.

Lois says: Despite my career as a beauty editor, I never wore real foundation. It may surprise you, but that's something many beauty editors have in common. I flirted with tinted moisturizer but basically I relied on a year-round tan (a real one until age thirty-five and then self-tanner) and bronzing powder for extra color and a little camouflage. Wearing foundation felt "old" and very un-cool. When I started seriously dealing with sun damage my view changed. Skin cancer and brown spots will do that. As a recovered foundation phobic, I've become a foundation junkie. It's become my most important cosmetic.

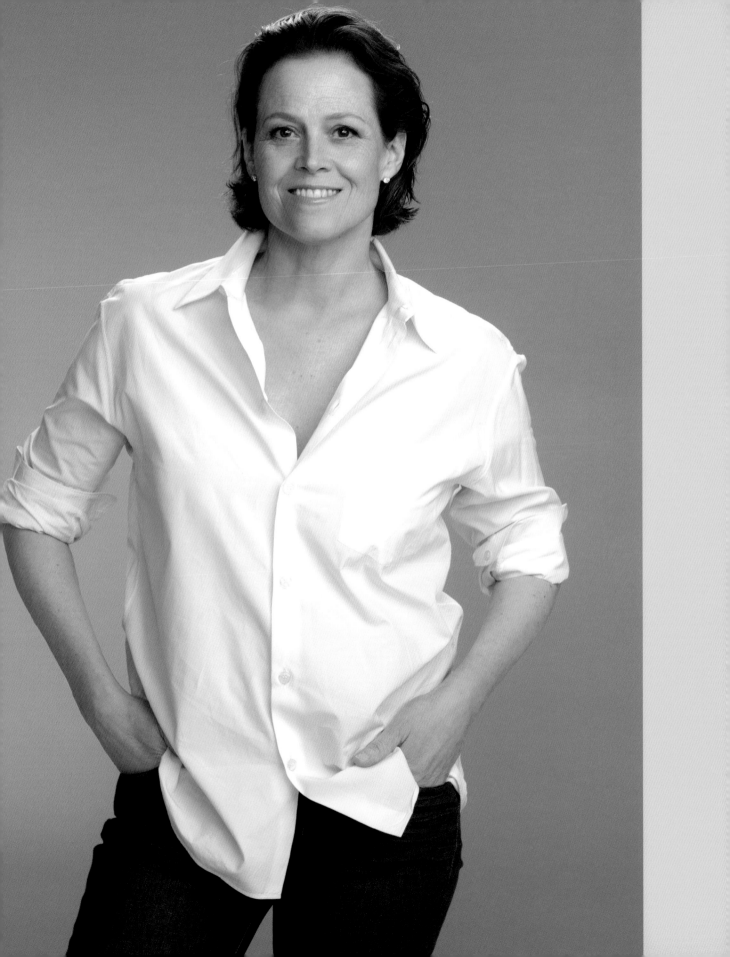

What the right face makeup can do for you now

Foundation can give you fresher, healthier-looking skin and minimize the look of sun damage in minutes. Don't get caught up in the long-term treatment aspects of foundation as your primary concern. And don't aim for flawless coverage or a chin to hairline even wash of color. That just looks like a mask. Sometimes little imperfections are welcome and actually make you look younger.

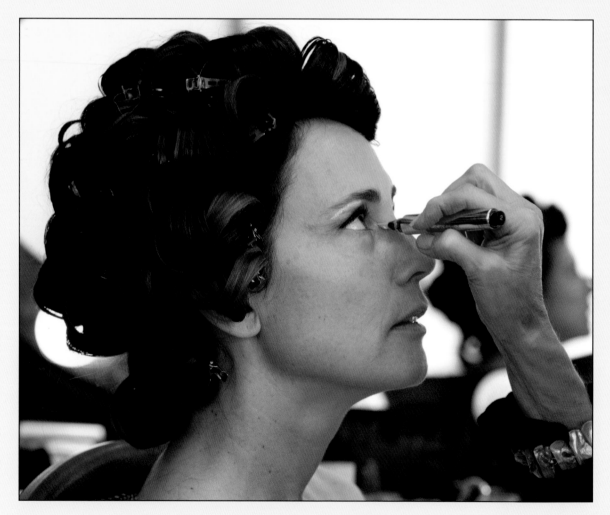

No-surgery Foundation

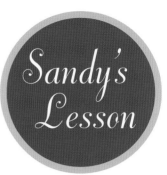

Sandy's Lesson

A lot of us got by on a minimal makeup look for decades. Others have followed a routine of foundation, concealer, and powder for years but it's not working anymore. Try it with my technique.

You'll need:

- moisturizer or sunscreen with treatment
- primer (optional)
- foundation
- foundation brush
- dense opaque concealer
- concealer brush
- makeup sponge
- pressed or loose powder (optional)
- highlighter pen (optional)

1 **Apply primer, moisturizer with an SPF, or sunscreen under your foundation—but avoid multiple layers of product!** You can't start your makeup by piggybacking sunscreen, treatment, moisturizer, serums, and primer and then expect great-looking foundation to follow. Use fewer products more efficiently and be selective. If you've had skin cancer or pre-cancers or spend a lot of time outdoors or in direct sunlight (in front of a glass office window, for example), of course you want to use a high SPF under your makeup. In that case choose a broad spectrum sunscreen that's makeup

compatible, in a moisturizing or matte formula, depending on your skin's needs. Primer can help smooth the surface so textural problems like lines, flakes, and pores don't interfere with makeup application. Save your heavy-duty repair skincare for bedtime.

Make your foundation work harder than your concealer for coverage. You may end up using more foundation and no concealer at all! It's an important switch because most women use more concealer than foundation. That's fine when you're young. Now you're dealing with a pasty complexion or sun damage, not just a few blemishes and circles. I use liquid foundation or a cream base in a compact on most clients and as little concealer as possible because the under eye area will look older with too much concealer or too much foundation. The key to avoiding a heavily made-up look is to vary and control the density during application. This means your foundation will be sheer in some areas and layered for coverage in others—not of equal weight or intensity all over the face.

Look for the right color first and then check for texture. Go deeper in foundation color and keep it warm in tone. Remember the rule about "test four shades on your jaw and the one that disappears is your match?" Forget it. Most women choose a shade that's too light. Go at least half a shade to one shade deeper in foundation color than you think. If a new client says she uses a #2 base, I usually boost her to a 2.5 or a 3—sometimes a 3.5! If you've been using the same shade for years you might be resistant to change at first. That's why when I'm working on a client and changing her shade I always start by sneaking it on at the jaw line, near the ear. The client can't see what I'm doing and this little trick allows me to get the base on before she can comment on the shade change. By the time I reach the nose she's happy.

When a foundation is warmer, a little on the yellow side, you look real. Pink-based foundation gives a fake "painted lady" effect no matter how well you apply it. Color matters more after forty-five because your skin tone goes through dramatic changes. You

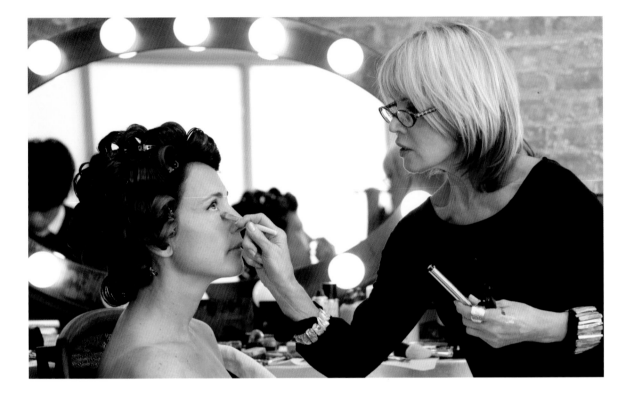

can always manipulate texture a little but you cannot manipulate color. Each brand has a rating system for its shades. Knowing what shade range you are makes selection easier. Avoid foundations categorized as cool and shade names like cool beige, fair, or rose beige, because they usually have pink undertones. Look for shades characterized as warm or with names that include the words warm, nude, honey, sandy, caramel, or golden. Makeup artist Bobbi Brown started the change to correctly promote yellow-based foundations. Head for a cosmetic counter and a brand known for its great foundations like Laura Mercier, Bobbi Brown, Lancôme, Estée Lauder, or M.A.C. for guidance.

 Test foundation twice—first by applying it to the back of your hand with a clenched fist and then on your cheek.
Make a fist and apply foundation to the back of your hand as if it's your face. When you open and relax your hand, the skin loosens and gives you a pretty accurate idea of how the makeup will react to expression lines, dryness, and saggy areas. From this test you can

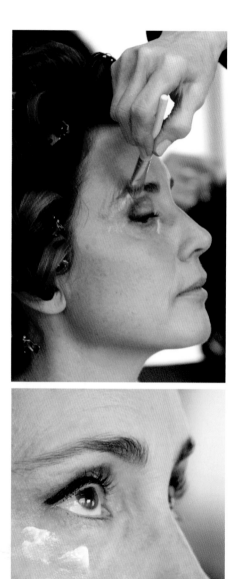

also tell how much coverage you can expect with brown spots. This trick can help you decide if the texture is too shimmery or too matte, too dry or too greasy, too sheer or too heavy. Then test the foundation for pore visibility. The right makeup should never make your pores more obvious. In fact, it should make them less obvious. Do this second test on the cheek area, where pores are usually smaller. If a foundation emphasizes pores there, it will never work on your T-zone where the pores are larger. Try both of these tests at home to evaluate foundations you already own before shopping for new ones.

5 Squirt or dab a drop of makeup at a time on the back of your non-working hand (left if you're a righty and vice versa). Work from the back of your hand, acting as a palette, using a foundation brush. I know it looks wasteful to non-pros but there are three practical reasons this works. One, you become more aware of how much makeup you are applying and can evaluate need as you go. Two, your body temperature warms the foundation so it goes on easily and smoothly without excess work. Three, you also actually see the texture and color of the product against your skin as you apply it.

6 **Use a quality foundation brush to apply foundation. It's what really makes the difference for skin that has lost its taut, firm feeling.** Look for foundation brushes with synthetic bristles. As a professional makeup artist I use everything from brushes to sponges to my fingers to blend and perfect makeup. Non-pros benefit from a good brush because they use less product, manipulate the texture more easily, and are able to blend it without leaving streaks or borderlines. Apply the foundation with a back and forth motion and use a beating or patting motion for extra coverage. Pat around the edges of the nose, upper cheeks, and between your nose and upper lip.

7 **Start around the edges of the face and blend inwards. Women usually start in the center of the face and forget to blend and feather the color out towards the edges.** Begin at the jaw and move the brush in quick strokes working up and in. Don't neglect the

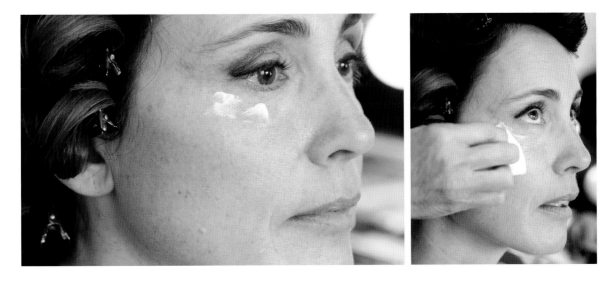

forehead, hairline, the seam where your ears meet your face, and under the jaw. If you're wearing bangs skip foundation on the forehead because you won't need the extra coverage there and all it will do is make your bangs greasy. Feather the edges down to where the neck starts. Brush against the grain of the skin where you have deep folds—from nose to mouth, for example. Resist applying foundation directly under your eyes, where the skin is thin and prone to crinkling.

8 **Use a damp latex makeup sponge to pat off excess and take away the makeup-y edge. Don't wipe, pat!** Sometimes I will decide to go sheerer in certain areas when I'm done. A damp wedge sponge skimmed over the face makes the foundation appear like real skin. You will never look like you're wearing foundation if you use this trick. It also helps blend makeup at the jaw line.

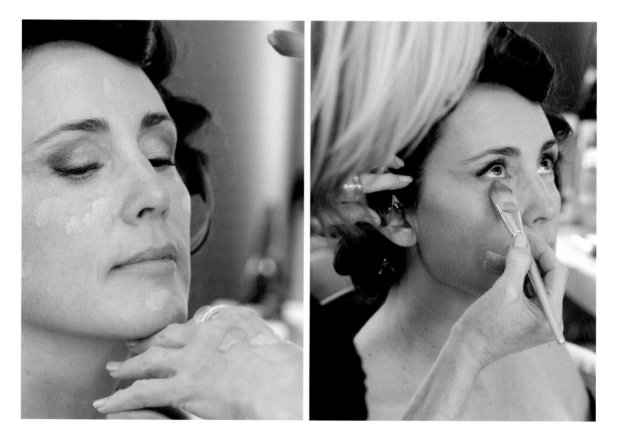

9 Try using foundation as "concealer" before adding real concealer. You need to be very discriminating. Apply full-coverage concealer on brown spots or dark circles only after you've used your foundation as much as possible for camouflage. You want to avoid applying too much concealer. Many women unnecessarily overdose on coverage in the eye area. I like creamy concealers like Clé de Peau Beauté Concealer and Lancôme Effacernes for extra eye coverage. At some point however, under eye concealer is useless. I opt not to use it on women with very thin skin under the eyes. Instead, I use a highlighter pen on the inner corner of the eyes or under the brow. The last thing we need is highlighted wrinkles. A soft white pencil is useful on the deep inner corner of the eye and will brighten the eye in place of concealer, which doesn't cut it anymore.

On brown spots, Dermablend Smooth Indulgence Concealer or CM-Beauty by Cover-mark Coverstik are excellent for full coverage. They are transfer resistant and do not move. To apply concealer, use a concealer brush to pick up a small amount of concealer and press it directly over the discoloration.

Use concealer sparingly. Don't move it around or try to blend it out. The idea is to control placement in a very specific way. Take a clean shadow brush and apply powder right over the concealer, pressing the bristles gently in place against the skin. Don't rub. Use a gentle touch so you don't remove any concealer. If your eyes are in pretty good shape you just need foundation.

10 Use powder on the face very sparingly, if at all. I rarely use powder on women for everyday wear anymore—skin looks fresher and more youthful without it! If you're just lost without powder, apply it in the T-zone and under your cheeks—not on top of them. Dust on a translucent loose powder if necessary using a brush or puff. Have a compact with you always for any necessary checkups or touchups.

I'm Obsessed with My...

Very thin "onion paper" skin: A sheer, very lightweight moisturizing foundation or a tinted moisturizer won't look heavy or sit on the surface of your skin. Use Sandy's damp sponge trick (page 104) to remove superficial excess from the surface once you're done.

Hormonal acne: The hygienic mist of an airbrush foundation can make spots, zits, and excess redness virtually disappear. New pod-type sprays are spin-offs of the bigger pro machines TV and film makeup artists have been using for years.

Serious brown spots: Very dark or large brown spots need opaque coverage that is transfer-resistant like Dermablend Smooth Indulgence Concealer or CM-Beauty by Covermark Coverstik. It will save you time.

For covering large areas try CM-Beauty by Covermark Classic Cover or Dermablend Professional Cover Creme Foundation SPF 30.

Splotchy red skin/Rosacea: A yellow-toned moisturizer counteracts redness and gives flushed skin a more uniform color without heavy allover coverage. Aim for a sunny glow, not a porcelain perfect look. Whatever you do, skip those ghastly green primers that claim to correct reddish skin tones. They are confusing! A product such as Sensual Skin Enhancer by Kevyn Aucoin, used with a concealer brush, really works.

Large pores on nose: Use a mattifying primer or a matte sunscreen before applying foundation. They absorb oil and give your skin a cleaner finish. Use a concealer brush in a back and forth and patting motion when applying makeup to this area.

Lasered reverse raccoon eyes: Under eye laser treatments can leave that area looking lighter than the rest of your face. Pop a little yellow concealer along the border where lasered skin meets your foundation. It takes the edge off and helps connect the two skin shades.

Super-dark circles: Get yourself a tinted corrective eye concealer like Laura Mercier Eye Perfecter. It comes in two deep intense shades, mauve/rose for brownish circles and orange/yellow for blue or purple circles. Use a concealer brush to apply.

Puffy upper lids: Apply a chilled eye treatment that contains either yeast complex, like Patricia Wexler M.D. Dermatology Fastscription Instant De-Puff Eye Gel, or caffeine, like Olay Professional Pro-X Eye Restoration Complex, to tighten the skin. Cold brings the swelling down faster so keep these in the fridge ready and waiting. Use a dark pencil liner over the lid and blend it in. Soften the pencil with a shadow brush and retrace the pencil line with a medium dark shadow. Blacks and browns work best.

face makeup

secrets of celebs and models 40+

Celebs get their foundation sprayed on! They sometimes request that the spray treatment done for TV and film appearances be done for events and parties too. Machines use pods of pigment, a compressor, and a hose to mist on foundation for allover total coverage and a perfectly even look.

Models learn to wear a high SPF sunscreen and a hat whether on vacation or a photo shoot. In addition to sun damage, tanning makes makeup application difficult.

Models check face makeup close up and four feet from the mirror. Makeup has to work at normal distances—the way others see you. Or, as our friend Lauren Ezersky says, "I do my makeup in an ordinary mirror—the only ones getting close enough to see my pores are my Chihuahuas and they don't care!" Remember no one sees you in a magnifying mirror but you!

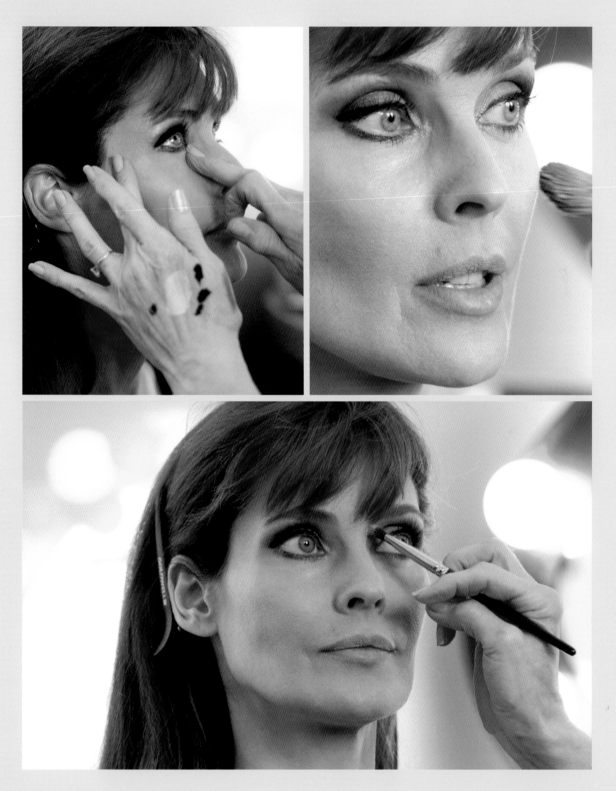

The Top Face Makeup Mistakes Most Women Make

Using color correctors. Tinted bases in mauve, pink, or pistachio green are one of the biggest makeup myths going. They don't cancel out blotchy skin or discolorations. They just add another layer of weird color to prevent your foundation from doing its job.

Choosing pink-based foundation after peels or laser treatment. Big mistake! The newly exposed skin is going to be shiny and pinker for a while (don't worry, that fades). Don't make it worse by using pink-based foundation. Instead, go warmer to compensate for the extra rosiness. Use a cream foundation because it will adhere to the skin.

Staying loyal to foundation you have used forever. If you're still wearing the same foundation color you wore in college make sure it's still right for you. Foundation should be warmer toned as you age.

Skipping foundation. Your forties or fifties may be the first time you really do need coverage. If you believe in growing old "gracefully"—and by that we mean going gray and nixing any dermatological help—a little foundation can make the difference between dowdy and delicious.

Double dipping with fingers.

Do not poke your finger in the bottle or jar and apply foundation, even if you've just washed your hands. It's the easiest way to get bacteria in the foundation and a roaring skin infection. Trust us. Medicinal steroids are not fun.

Using shimmery foundation on a full face.
Women with full faces should avoid shimmery or dewy "radiance boosting" foundation. They make faces look wider and plumper. Matte foundation is preferable.

Not using a real makeup remover at night.
There is no way you can have great-looking skin without using a makeup remover. Some soaps, mousses, and gels are perfect for light morning washing but really won't get all the makeup pigment out of your pores.

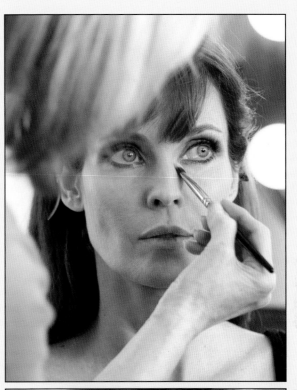

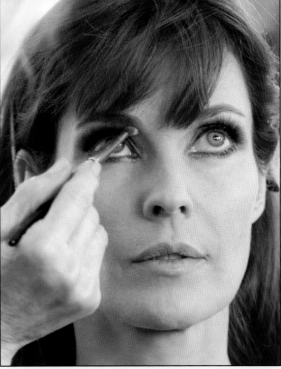

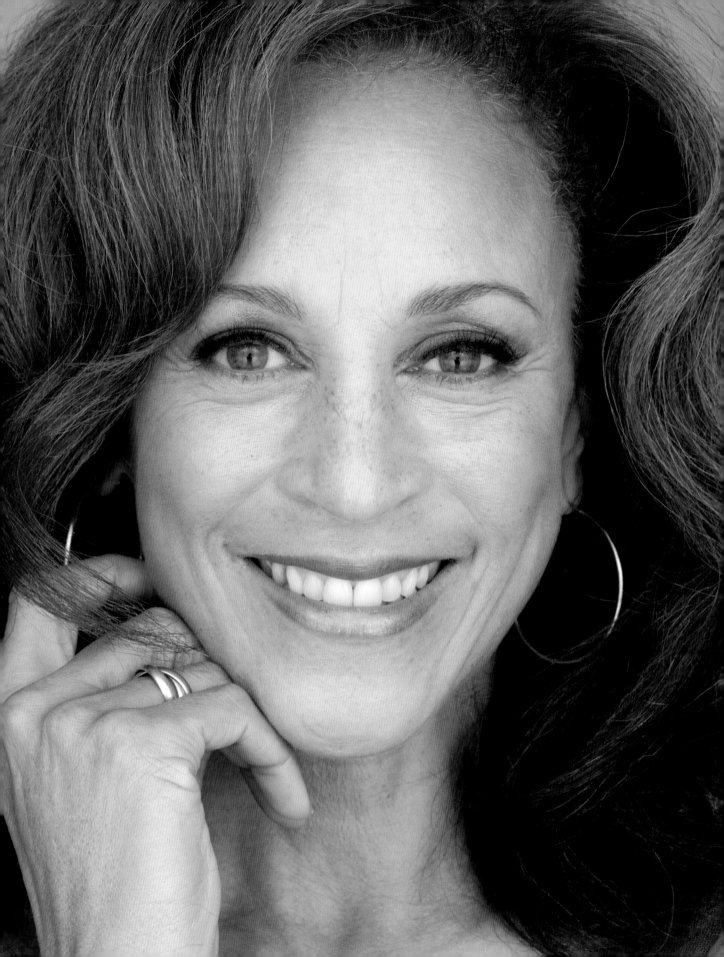

Alva Chinn

"I never used to wear makeup when I wasn't in front of the camera or on a runway, but now that I'm in my fifties I need to do some corrective makeup to feel my best. Under eye concealer for me is a big must. I use a peachy color and then I use a tiny bit of foundation to blend it into the rest of my skin. I add some blush, mascara, and a little definition around my eyes and brows. A little makeup makes me look younger now.

I have naturally dark circles under my eyes that looked cool when I was younger but I correct them now.

My skin tone changes dramatically depending on the season and I have freckles. I'm golden brown-coppery in summer, green beige in winter, and my forehead is darker around the edges. I need a warm base and I still mix foundations to get what I want. I go deeper in foundation in winter; lighter in summer. I use a mineral powder makeup that is professionally mixed."

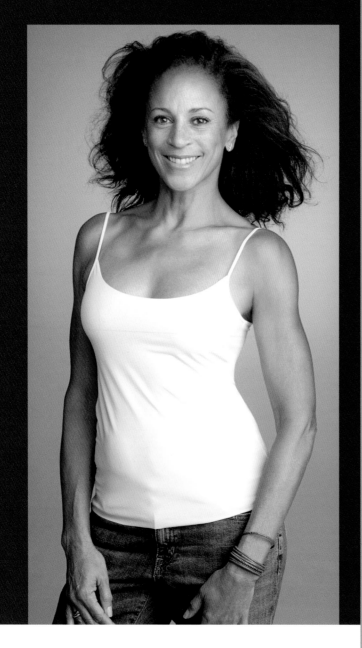

Take your makeup blending into account when wearing a top or dress with a low neckline. The transition from face to neck to chest should be seamless.

PROS+CONS

We have our own favorites when it comes to face makeup. My experience as a beauty editor and serious former sun worshipper and Sandy's as a makeup artist and former average tanner, plus our own personal preferences, mimic exactly what real women we work with say and think. Here's where we differ and why.

Q: Foundation. Drugstore or department store brands?
Liquid, cream, or powder base?

Sandy says: I honestly don't use or wear drugstore foundation. It comes down to not having the chance to test it first. Clients who do like a certain drugstore foundation tell me the shade they want is often hard to find. I find the stock is just not as reliable in drugstores as department stores. There's no beauty advisor at hand to help you special order your shade or help you make the transition to another formula if a line is discontinued. I love liquids, cream compacts, and spray-ons, but I try everything new that catches my eye. Everyday clients give the best feedback on how well a specific foundation performs. In the studio I'm constantly monitoring and adjusting the makeup on set.

I stopped using cream foundations that come in jars when I dropped a heavy glass one on the floor of Jessica Lange's hotel room. Cleaning up the mess cured me of carting them around in my kit. Thick, whipped foundations like those are also psychologically unappealing to a lot of women.

As a beauty editor I get to sample new makeup from every brand—high end and low. Some pricey foundations really have qualities that merit a splurge, but I'm also a genuine fan of low-cost foundations from CoverGirl and L'Oréal Paris. I apply a liquid or cream base at home and carry a stick foundation or cream compact for touchups. Try on new foundations bare-faced and make it a project for a free morning when stores are less crowded. Whip on a big pair of sexy sunglasses and go without makeup to a department store or Sephora. Take along all your "mistakes" for comparison.

● ●

Q ● **Concealer. High-coverage or light-reflecting wands?**
● **Skin-tone shades or tinted bisques, peaches, and apricots?**

I like three kinds of concealer. First a stick one for the under eye area like Clé de Peau or tubes like Lancôme Effacernes. I like a thick opaque crème concealer to counteract excess pigment in brown spots and deep discolorations. This concealer should really stick to the skin and be transfer resistant like those by Dermablend or CM-Beauty by Covermark. A highlighter pen like the tinted shimmery YSL Touche Éclat is the other essential. It adds sparkle to tired eyes and can be layered on later in the day for touchups.

Like most former sun tanners I have big coverage issues due to extensive sun damage. Opaque concealers in peachy tones and shimmery pink highlighter are everyday basics—I'd give up mascara and blush before I'd let go of these. I depend on #2 YSL Touche Éclat, Bobbi Brown Corrector in Light Bisque, Clé de Peau Beauté Concealer in Ivory, and Laura Mercier's Secret Camouflage in SC-2, plus foundation when I need to look fresh. No kidding—all five.

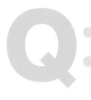 **Q:** **To powder or not to powder?**

 Sandy says: I hardly use powder anymore to set makeup or blot shine and when I do it's minimal—just lightly in the T-zone if the skin requires it. Some foundations are so thin though, that they need translucent powder to adhere to the skin.

 Lois says: Guerlain Meteorites Powder for the Face and I go way back. These pea-sized multicolor balls of powder come in a round box that looks like something from Marie Antoinette's dressing table and they smell like violets. You swirl your

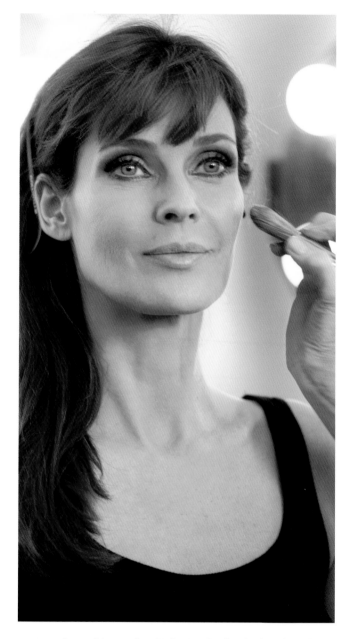

brush in them and apply all over your face. I love the Pink Fresh shade for the sheer golden glow it adds over foundation with no cakey, powdery look.

I've tried mineral powder foundation for summer or travel to humid climates, but I'm very picky and can't say I actually prefer it to fluid foundation. I think powder foundation on its own just exacerbates dryness and lines.

EXPERIENCE

- **Wash your foundation and concealer brushes to keep them fluffy, silky, and clean.** Use a special makeup brush cleanser or shampoo. Plain old soap and water will make the bristles spiky when they dry. Rinse thoroughly to press out excess water and reshape the bristles. Let the brush head hang over the edge of your sink to dry so air gets to the hairs and fluffs them out.

- **Some women prefer a tinted moisturizer.** That's fine, but select one with the right texture and shade options. A one-size-fits-all tinted moisturizer isn't going to do anything.

- **If you like a powdery finish but don't want to wear powder,** try a semi-matte primer, a velvety semi-matte foundation, or a sheer matte liquid.

- **If you spent money on a luxurious new foundation but find it still isn't perfect,** try applying a clear silicone primer to "correct" texture.

- **All brushes are not the same.** Brushes for wet products, like foundation and concealer, are different from those for dry products, like powder blush. Ask for them by name.

Constance White

"Makeup is a much healthier, more affordable, more accessible alternative to plastic surgery. For me a big change that came with age is that I wear makeup four out of seven days a week. Ten years ago I'd wear makeup maybe one day out of seven. I've stopped buying into the wrinkle cream of the minute. I do a moisturizer with sunblock for day, a moisturizer at night, and some Vaseline; I use Vitamin E oil or botanical oil around my eyes; Kiehl's lip balm—especially in winter. When I started to do TV for my work as Style Director for eBay, I was exposed to more makeup experts and their artistry. I learned never to go on camera without makeup. The naked eye sees things very differently than the camera. Off-camera I can now do my makeup in five minutes flat—and in a moving vehicle! Another thing TV and exposure to makeup artists did for me is influence me to take better care of my skin. I always cleanse with a gentle cleanser, moisturize, and treat my breakouts (yeah, I still get them). And now I see a dermatologist at least twice a year. I still prefer light makeup but technically I need a yellow-toned warm foundation and powder. I use mostly Black Opal but also Bobbi Brown, M.A.C., Cynde Watson, and YSL. I look for foundation that matches my skin tone first and then a powder to matte my skin down a bit. I seek out informed saleswomen at the counter though I find makeup artists give better information."

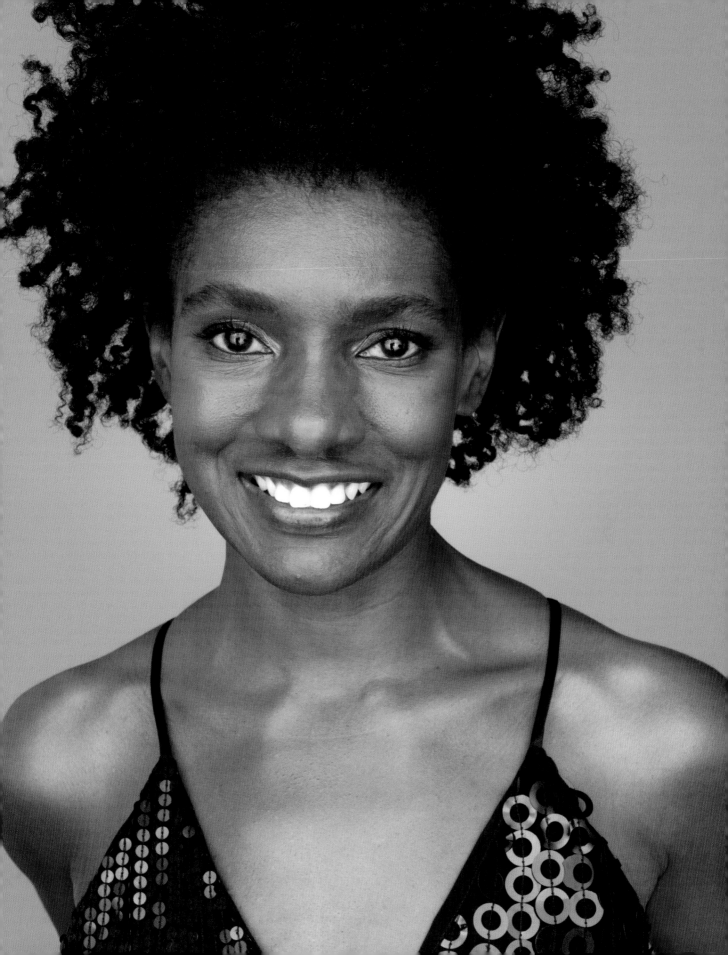

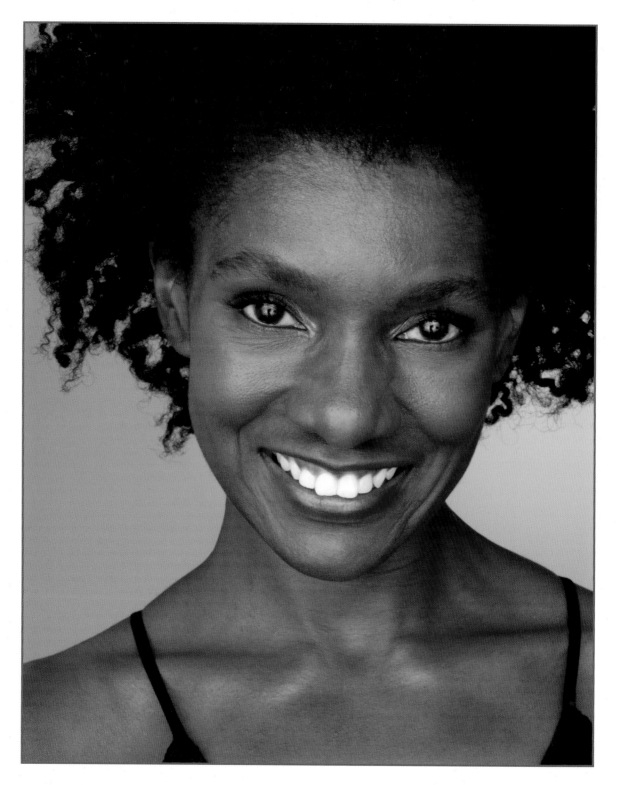

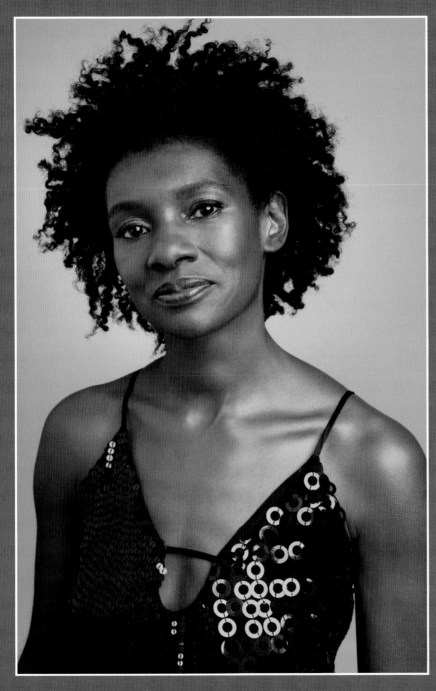

Sandy + Lois TIP

Most women have variations in their face and body skin tone. Choose a foundation that blends the two and then add a healthy pop of cheek color for a more even effect.

The beauty stalkers

Exfoliators

Smooth away dead cells and flakes for better makeup application. Speed up cell turnover with an at-home peel, polishing scrub, or enzyme mask as part of your skincare routine. We suggest:

- **Clé de Peau Beauté Micro-Refining Treatment** ($200 neimanmarcus.com)
- **Dr. Patricia Wexler M.D. Dermatology Sensitive Skin Gentle Exfoliating Peel** ($35 bathandbodyworks.com)
- **Erno Laszlo C-Peel** ($75 ernolaszlo.com)
- **ExfoliKate by Kate Somerville** ($65 sephora.com)
- **Kiehl's Since 1851 Pineapple Papaya Facial Scrub** ($26 kiehls.com)
- **Olay Regenerist Thermal Mini-Peel** ($26 drugstores)
- **Lancôme Exfoliant Fraichelle** ($31.50 lancome-usa.com)

Daily moisturizers with sunscreen

To protect and hydrate your skin under makeup:

- **La Mer The SPF 30 UV Protecting Fluid** ($65 cremedelamer.com) **formulated to be used over . . .**
- **La Mer The Moisturizing Lotion** ($190 cremedelamer.com)
- **Lancôme Absolue Premium Bx Absolute Replenishing Cream SPF 15** ($125 lancome-usa.com)
- **La Roche-Posay Anthelios SX Daily Moisturizing Cream with Sunscreen SPF 15** ($29.95 laroche-posayus.com)
- **Neutrogena Healthy Defense Daily Moisturizer SPF 30 with PureScreen** ($13 drugstores)

go shopping for

Face Products

- Dr. Patricia Wexler MD Dermatology Sensitive Skin Calming Anti-Aging Moisturizer SPF 30 ($39.50 bathandbodyworks.com)

Makeup compatible sunscreens

If you prefer starting your makeup with a true sunscreen, try these:

- Clinique Super City Block Oil-Free Daily Face Protector SPF 40 ($17.50 clinique.com)

- Neutrogena Ultra Sheer Liquid Sunblock Fluid SPF 55 with Helioplex ($12 drugstores)

- Dr. Brandt UV SPF 30 High Protection Face Tinted or Untinted ($35 drbrandtskincare.com)

- La Roche-Posay Anthelios 40 with Mexoryl SX Sunscreen ($32 laroche-posayus.com)

Pore smoothing primers

Gently spackle these primers to smooth pores on your nose prior to foundation:

- Clé de Peau Beauté Smoothing Base for Pores SPF 24 ($75 neimanmarcus.com)

- Lancôme La Base Pro ($42 lancome-usa.com)

- Clinique Pore Minimizer Instant Perfector ($17.50 clinique.com)

- Dr. Brandt Pores No More Refiner ($45 drbrandtskincare.com)

- Yves Saint Laurent Matt Touch Pre-Makeup Base ($42 saksfifthavenue.com)

Dry skin primers

Makes thin dry skin feel like cushy velvet:

- **Dr. Patricia Wexler M.D. Dermatology MMPi.20 Skin Regenerating Serum**

  ($150 bathandbodyworks.com)

- **L'Oréal Paris Studio Secrets Professional Magic Perfecting Base**

  ($10.99 drugstores)

- **La Prairie Cellular Treatment Rose Illusion Line Filler** ($115 neimanmarcus.com)

Foundations

For extra hydration plus coverage:

- **Bobbi Brown Luminous Moisturizing Foundation** ($45 bobbibrowncosmetics.com)
- **Chanel Vitalumière Moisture-Rich Radiance Fluid Makeup SPF 15** ($54 chanel.com)
- **Dior Diorskin Nude Natural Glowing Hydrating Makeup** ($46 sephora.com)
- **Estée Lauder Nutritious Vita-Mineral Makeup SPF 10** ($34 esteelauder.com)
- **Giorgio Armani Designer Shaping Cream Foundation SPF 20**

  ($65 giorgioarmanibeauty-usa.com)

- **Guerlain Parure Gold Fluid Foundation** ($78 neimanmarcus.com)
- **Lancôme Teinte Miracle** ($37 lancome-usa.com)

Weightless coverage for thin, fine-textured skin:

- **Chanel Lift Lumière Firming and Smoothing Fluid Makeup SPF 15**

  ($65 chanel.com)

- **Kevyn Aucoin The Liquid Airbrush Foundation** ($45 kevynaucoin.com)
- **L'Oréal Paris True Match Super Blendable Makeup** ($6.99 drugstores)
- **NARS Sheer Glow Foundation** ($42 narscosmetics.com)
- **Stila Illuminating Liquid Foundation** ($38 stilacosmetics.com)
- **Trish McEvoy Treatment Foundation SPF 15** ($75 nordstrom.com)

Extra coverage that's not heavy or masky for sun-damaged skin
with extreme pigmentation issues:

- **Bobbi Brown Stick Foundation** ($40 bobbibrowncosmetics.com)
- **Clé de Peau Beauté Refining Fluid Foundation SPF 24** ($118 neimanmarcus.com)
- **Giorgio Armani Face Fabric Foundation SPF 12** ($48 giorgioarmanibeauty-usa.com)
- **Laura Mercier Silk Crème Foundation** ($42 lauramercier.com)
- **Make Up For Ever HD Invisible Cover Foundation** ($40 sephora.com)
- **M.A.C. Select SPF 15 Mineralize Foundation** ($32 maccosmetics.com)

Long-wear bases that hot-flash proof the skin:

- **Clinique Even Better Makeup SPF 15** ($24.50 clinique.com)
- **Estée Lauder Double Wear Light Stay-In-Place Makeup SPF 10** ($34 esteelauder.com)
- **Giorgio Armani Lasting Silk UV Foundation SPF 20** ($59 giorgioarmanibeauty-usa.com)

Tinted moisturizers

Moisture plus light color for thin, spotted, sun-damaged skin:

- **La Mer The SPF 18 Fluid Tint** ($65 cremedelamer.com)
- **Lancôme Bienfait Multi-Vital Teinté High Potency Tinted Moisturizer Vitamin Enriched UVA/UVB SPF 30** ($45 lancome-usa.com)
- **Laura Mercier Tinted Moisturizer SPF 20** ($42 sephora.com)
- **M.A.C. Studio Moisture Tint SPF 15** ($29.50 maccosmetics.com)
- **Stila Sheer Color Tinted Moisturizer SPF 15** ($34 stilacosmetics.com)

Spray-on foundations

For multiple pigmentation issues and skin prone to hormonal breakouts:

- **DiorSkin Airflash Spray Foundation** ($60 sephora.com)
- **The Temptu Airbrush Makeup System** ($225 sephora.com)

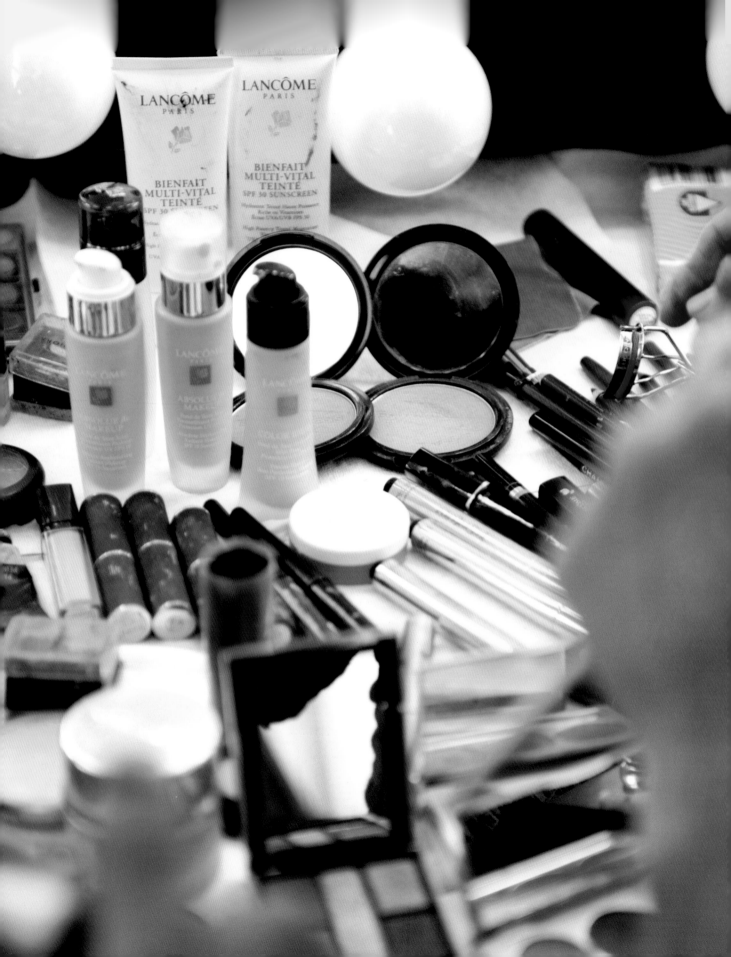

Portable touchups

Quick fixes for your bag:

- **Lancôme Photogenic Lumessence Compact** ($42 lancome-usa.com)

- **Bobbi Brown Face Touch-Up Stick** ($22 bobbibrowncosmetics.com)

- **CoverGirl & Olay Simply Ageless Foundation** ($13.99 drugstores)

- **M.A.C. Studio Tech Foundation** ($29.50 maccosmetics.com)

- **Shiseido Makeup Advanced Hydro-Liquid Compact SPF 15** ($29.50 refill, $10.50 case, nordstrom.com)

Concealers

For covering everyday light to medium circles:

- **Lancôme Maquicomplet, all shades, particularly Correcteur** ($28.50 lancome-usa.com)

- **Bobbi Brown Tinted Eye Brightener** ($38 bobbibrowncosmetics.com)

- **Chanel Lift Lumière Concealer** ($45 chanel.com)

- **Edward Bess Platinum Concealer** ($38 edwardbess.com)

- **Lancôme Effacernes Undereye Concealer** ($28.50 lancome-usa.com)

- **Laura Mercier Secret Concealer** ($22 lauramercier.com)

- **M.A.C. Studio Sculpt Concealer** ($16.50 maccosmetics.com)

For coverage of light brown spots, blemishes, and spider veins:

- **Clé de Peau Beauté Concealer** ($70 neimanmarcus.com)

- **Laura Mercier Secret Camouflage** ($28 sephora.com)

- **Make Up For Ever Full Cover Concealer** ($30 sephora.com)

For covering very dark or multiple brown spots:

- **CM-Beauty by Covermark Coverstik** ($15 cm-beauty.com)

- **CM-Beauty by Covermark Face Magic** ($17 cm-beauty.com)

- **Dermablend Professional Cover Creme Foundation SPF 30** ($32 dermablend.com)

- **Dermablend Smooth Indulgence Concealer** ($21 dermablend.com)

- **Kryolan Dermacolor Mini Palette 71006** ($34.99 stageandtheatermakeup.com)

For covering very dark under-eye circles:

- **Bobbi Brown Corrector** ($22 bobbibrowncosmetics.com)
- **Laura Mercier Under Eye Perfecter** ($22 lauramercier.com)

For brightening fatigued eyes:

- **Yves Saint Laurent Touche Éclat Radiant Touch Highlighter** ($40 sephora.com)

Powders

- **Guerlain Meteorites Powder for the Face, in Pink Fresh, Beige Chic**
  ($56 sephora.com)
- **Kevyn Aucoin The Gossamer Loose Powder, in Diaphanous, Radiant Diaphanous**
  ($62 kevynaucoin.com)
- **Lancôme Absolue Powder Radiant Smoothing Powder** ($53 lancome-usa.com)
- **Lancôme Dual Finish Versatile Powder Makeup** ($35.50 lancome-usa.com)
- **Laura Mercier Mineral Finishing Powder** ($32 lauramercier.com)

Foundation and concealer brushes

For applying foundation:

- **Clinique Foundation Brush** ($32.50 clinique.com)
- **Dior Foundation Brush** ($32 saksfifthavenue.com)
- **La Mer The Foundation Brush** ($40 cremedelamer.com)
- **Lancôme Foundation Brush, #2** ($33.50 lancome-usa.com)
- **M.A.C. Foundation Brush, #190** ($32 maccosmetics.com)
- **M.A.C. Face Brush, #189** ($42 maccosmetics.com)
- **Make Up For Ever HD Brush, 30N** ($38 sephora.com)
- **Sephora Collection Retractable Foundation Brush, #56** ($24 sephora.com)
- **Shu Uemura Synthetic Brush, #14** ($40 shuuemura-usa.com)

For covering broken capillaries and blemishes or applying concealer in the eye area:

- **Bobbi Brown Concealer Brush** ($25 bobbibrowncosmetics.com)
- **Giorgio Armani Concealer Brush** ($36 giorgioarmanibeauty-usa.com)
- **Lancôme Concealer Brush, #8** ($25.50 lancome-usa.com)
- **Laura Mercier Secret Camouflage Brush** ($26 lauramercier.com)
- **Trish McEvoy M44 Precision Concealer Brush** ($25 nordstrom.com)
- **Alison Raffaele Concealer Brush Duo** ($27 alisonraffaele.com)

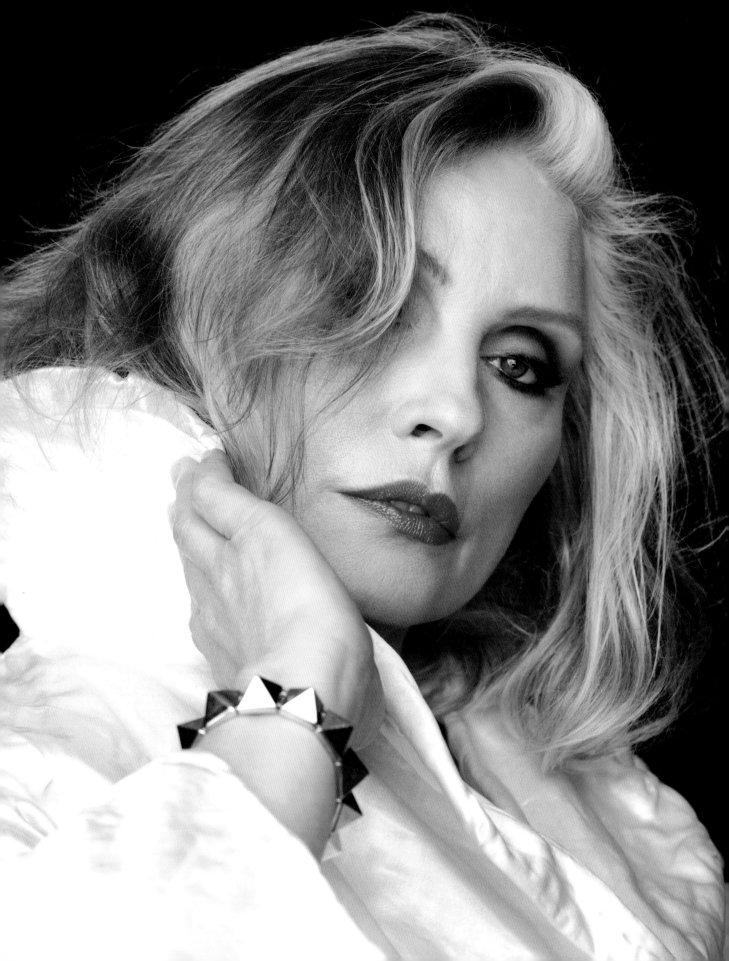

CHAPTER FOUR

GLOW, CHEEKBONES, AND SEXY LIPS

Blush and lipstick are the mood boosters of your makeup kit. The minute they're on we feel happier, brighter, and sexier. Blush and a shot of color on the lips make us feel upbeat. Color makes makeup a party, and for us, cheeks and lips are the perfect location. They're where we take advantage of our ability to swivel from bronzers to blushers, from gloss to full-on lipstick. The fun unravels when these features get stuck in a rut, because blush and lip colors date more quickly than any other makeup.

Deborah Harry

Grown-up Cheeks and Lips

Can you handle bad news? We have two things to tell you. First of all, your "apples"—the round, full part of the cheeks where blush used to go when you smiled—are no longer front and center. They've sagged and dropped lower on your face due to collagen, elastin, and fat loss. And sorry, second big newsflash: your lips have deflated and shrunk in size. They may look flat, thin, or asymmetrical. The lip border is probably faded and less defined and so is your natural lip color.

Change in your makeup application is mandatory. If you stick to the "apples" routine for blush placement, your cheek color will end up too far down. All you'll be doing is emphasizing the deep furrow called the nasolabial fold that runs from your nose to lips on either side of your mouth. Your thinned lips may now disappear completely when you smile and give your mouth a hard, pursed look. On the upside, the right makeup can easily and swiftly counteract these changes, starting today!

Find your new cheeks. Then put back some color. Shape your lips back in. This chapter will make you glow.

What was I thinking? Or, My Life in Blush, Bronzer, and Lipstick

We've been there with you.

In the 1990s, Ultima II launched The Nakeds and Bobbi Brown ignited a trend for beige and brown lipstick. Women breathed a sigh of relief. Neutrals gave makeup a badly needed makeover. What started as a trend grew into the go-to palette for everyday wear. Neutrals for lips and cheeks were easy to use and gave us a polished look for work, but allowed us to experiment and play with makeup in a confident way. Mistakes were nearly impossible. How can you overdo taupe, beige, and brown? The shades changed each year, adding more color diversity and texture options. Matte neutrals, our original safety zone in this category, began to shimmer and shine. Even our bronzers transitioned to improved formulas.

Makeup trends continue to shift all the time on the runway as fashion and the entertainment industry push beauty to extremes. We might see black glittery eyes and metallic cheeks and inky dark lips going mainstream for the twenty-something crowd, or pale matte lips and white eye shadow with big bold brows. Pay attention to what's going on. Know what's new but don't follow trends in an effort to look younger or hipper. Looking fresh, defined, and polished is what counts now.

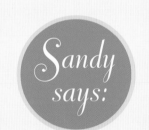

I think adding subtle color at a certain point starts looking more youthful than extremes like dark red or pale beige. I change my lip color from day to day and within the same day. More often than not I wear colored gloss over lip pencil. Soft pinks, mauves, roses, berry shades, and browns can be very flattering, especially in glosses or sheer lipsticks. When it comes to blush, I'm a big believer in its restorative power. It gives the face life.

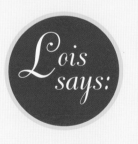

As a beauty editor and makeup minimalist I wore nude lips and cheeks for years—what Sandy jokingly calls my "invisible make-up." Now I feel cream blush or a shimmery powder in a pinky apricot color is the ultimate brightener. Under Sandy's influence I've finally moved on from beige to rosy pinks and golden peaches. She's right (although I resisted for a long time)—a little more color does wake you up after a certain age.

What the right cheeks and lips can do for you now

Blush makes you glow. Lip color gives you back definition.

Glow is what to aim for and it's a word that gets thrown around a lot. Everyone wants it but no one's sure how to get it. Sandy says glow is "the result of the way your skin reacts to makeup. It's the luminous, dewy quality, or healthy effect, that a product provides. A cream blush that turns dry, dull skin dewy gives you a glow; so does a slightly shimmery bronzer. Glow is what we are all trying to achieve when we apply makeup.

Lipsticks are just plain seductive—they're like candy and we get caught up in the thrill of improved textures, new shades, or (caution!) simply gorgeous packaging. Your lips can get a fresher and more youthful look with lip makeup in one of three ways:

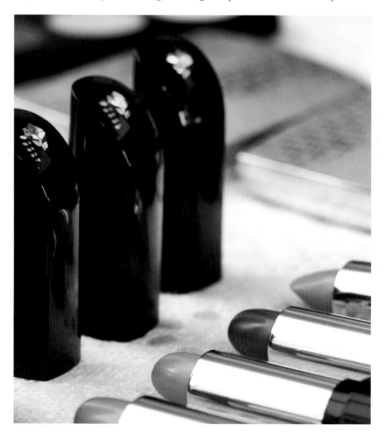

- If you're stuck on neutrals, upgrade your favorite to a shade with a hint more color.
- Soften bright lipsticks by switching to a sheer formula.
- Add gloss to your lipstick.

Whichever way you go, remember dark lipstick is not for you—no matter how edgy it looks on twenty-something models.

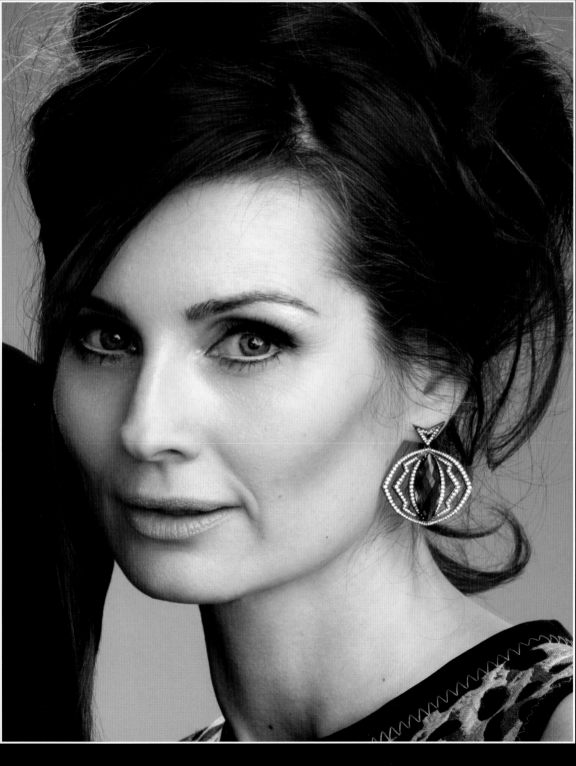

Jane Powers

"I love my forties. They seem to come with an inner self-confidence—in my opinions, my experiences, and my choices. Now confidence is totally an inside job and I'm in a good place. I have the life that I want and the love of my life, my son William. I can't say I look better than I did in my twenties, but I'm more comfortable with my looks and comfortable in my own skin. I've never dyed my hair and I have some beautiful expression lines that are just part of who I am."

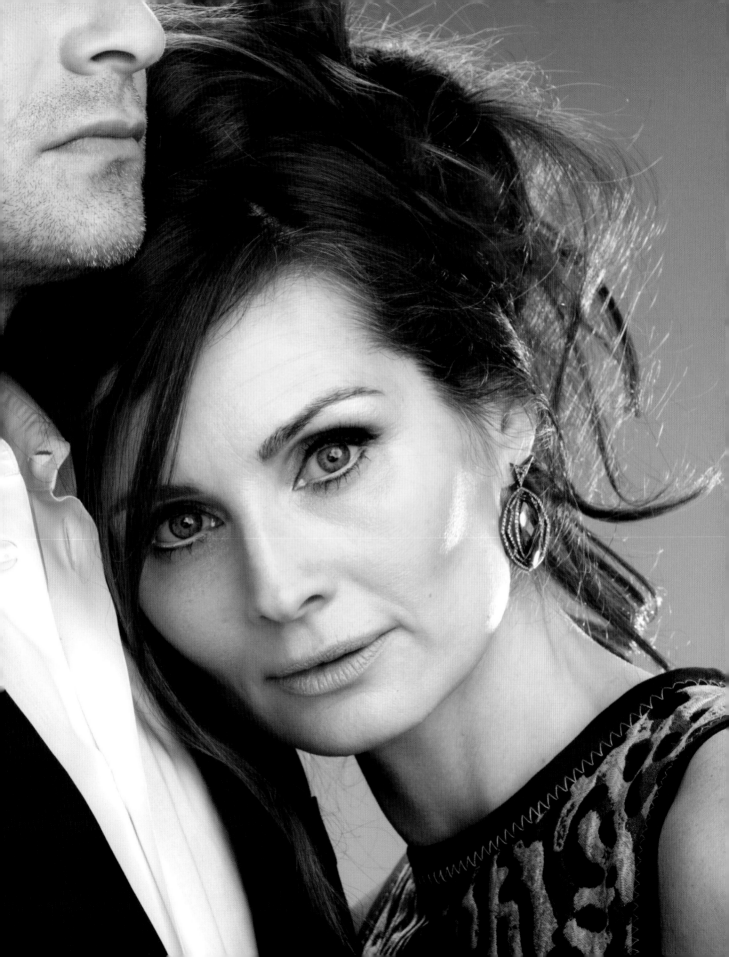

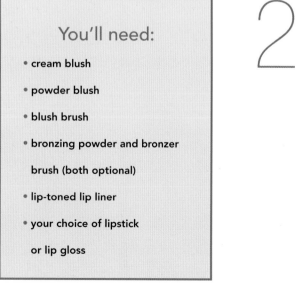

No-surgery Cheeks and Lips

1 **Take a good look at your face so far. You've done eyes, foundation, and concealer. You need balance.** Here's a general guideline for what's next. If you've emphasized your eyes with liner and shadow, you're going to want to keep lips low key. If your eye makeup is softer and/or your lips are your favorite feature, you might want to add more color on your mouth. Of course, highly spirited and very confident women can disregard this advice. I myself always apply eyes, lips, and cheeks of equal strength.

You'll need:

- **cream blush**
- **powder blush**
- **blush brush**
- **bronzing powder and bronzer brush (both optional)**
- **lip-toned lip liner**
- **your choice of lipstick or lip gloss**

2 **Add cream blush, powder blush, or a combo of both.** Skipping blush is out of the question, even if you use bronzing powder. The exceptions to this are women with the darkest skin tones. The texture you select is important. I think cream blush is amazing on dry skin and makes older skin bloom. For evening or a more pulled-together face I'll sometimes boost the color by adding a matching powder blush right over the cream blush.

Or I'll do the reverse and add a dab of cream blush over powder blush, or add bronzer using a light touch. Some women prefer a powder blush because it's quicker. Now that most of these powder formulas are sheer and moisturizing you don't have to worry about your blush looking dry or cakey.

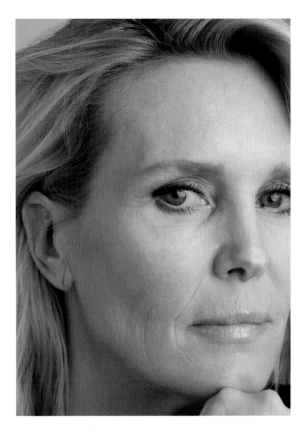

3 **Pink, apricot, or berry blushers energize your skin. They may look bright in the compact but once applied they add realistic warmth.** As always, texture and color matter. Look for clear colors in pink, apricot, coral, rose, or raspberry. The new formulas are highly pigmented but sheer in both cream and powder variations. Cream blush should be velvety, not greasy or dry, and blend on and into the skin easily. Powder blusher should have a silky texture and a lasting quality.

4 **If you wear bronzing powder you still need blush.** Even for women addicted to bronzer, blush has made a big comeback. The brightness of the color of the blush wakes up the face and makes the bronzer look more natural.

5 **No more applying blush to the apples of your cheeks (for most of you)! Move your blush high up to your cheekbones.** This is a major switch that changes everything. Decades ago, super-

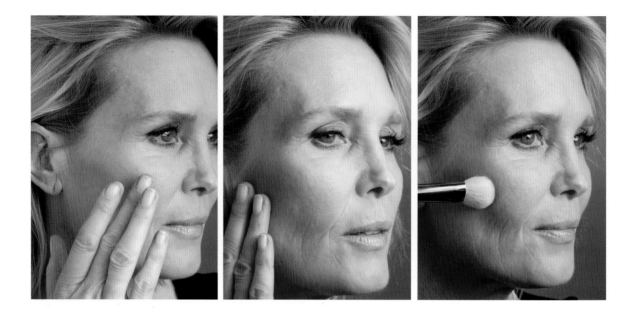

model Dayle Haddon taught me this trick. I still use it on Dayle and every single client. This is your new blush application. Look straight ahead into a mirror. Tap your cream blush along the cheekbone and over the cheekbone ledge. This brings back a look of bone structure and also keeps the emphasis on your eyes. You want to keep the color high on your cheekbone, not close to the nose or nasolabial folds.

6 If you're using powder blush, apply with a really big brush. The bigger the brush, the more finely the color will be dispersed on the skin so you just glow. If you use powder blush, the placement is the same—high on the cheekbone, not the apples. You may want to try using a really big powder brush instead of a standard blush brush. A blush brush that's too small will apply color too densely. Shake or tap off any excess on the back of your hand, then look straight ahead into a mirror and apply the blush under your pupil and along the cheekbone. Never turn your head to apply blush—you'll end up positioning the color too low on your face.

7 If you're using powder blush, let your under layer of moisturizer and foundation thoroughly set before applying the powder blush. That's the real reason powder blush streaks. I see women swirl their blush brush in powder blush and apply it immediately to skin still moist from foundation. Every time you use the brush again, the damp residue will make your powder blush cake and streak.

8 Use a natural-toned lip pencil that matches your lip color to correct asymmetries in the shape of your mouth. Lip liner quickly evens out a top lip that is lower or less defined on one side. This is one of the most common complaints I hear. If you have no bow anymore in your top lip, aim for a subtle rounded shape instead of drawing on two clearly fake peaks. Forget about using lip pencil to create the look of bigger lips by expanding the line past the border—it will just look fake.

Select a lip pencil shade that matches your own lip color as closely as possible. Use a very light touch and sketch along the weaker edge to balance it with the other. Then, color in the entire lip with the pencil. This provides a perfect base for any shade of lip gloss. A gloss over nude pencil is an easy way to work with a trendy or bright color.

Caution: If you have used any filler in your lips, you won't need lip liner to enhance size—you'll only over-emphasize what's already been done surgically.

9 Keep your favorite lip color, but switch up the texture and intensity. I tell women with thin lips who love real color to go sheerer in texture or softer in color. It's a good way to still keep the lips vibrant if your lips have thinned with age. Stay away from dark blue reds and burgundy shades that can give you a harsh look. For women who love the look of a nude lip, I suggest lining and filling in the entire lip with nude or lip-toned pencil, and then adding gloss on top.

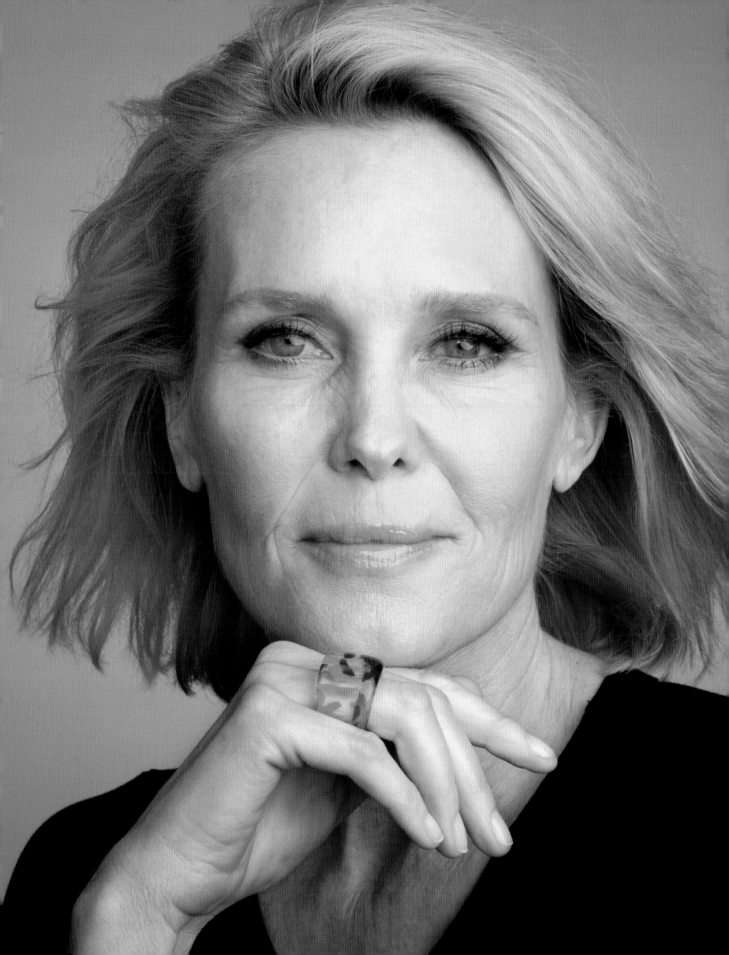

Nancy Donahue

"I love makeup. I won't go out of the house without concealer, blush, eyeliner, and mascara. When you hit your fifties, you need to put yourself together more. Maybe I'm a little vainer now that I'm fifty-two. I go for the fashion brands like Chanel Vitalumière foundation and Lancôme Teint Miracle foundation. I like high-end shadows, especially those by NARS. When it comes to skincare, although they're pricey, I use the Chanel cream, eye cream, and serum. My skin is Irish fair and fragile so I have to be careful about dermatological procedures, but I do go for Thermage and Vitamin C facials. I've developed a product called the HoneyBelle Bodybuffer and added that to my routine. It exfoliates every last flake, diminishes cellulite, and soothes sore muscles all in one go." (You can find the HoneyBelle Bodybuffer at bellebodybuffer.com)

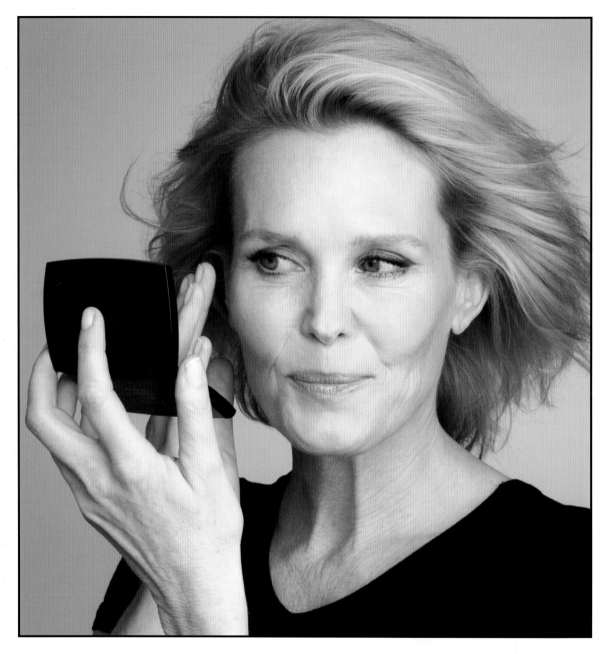

Applying blush high on the cheekbones draws attention to the eyes.

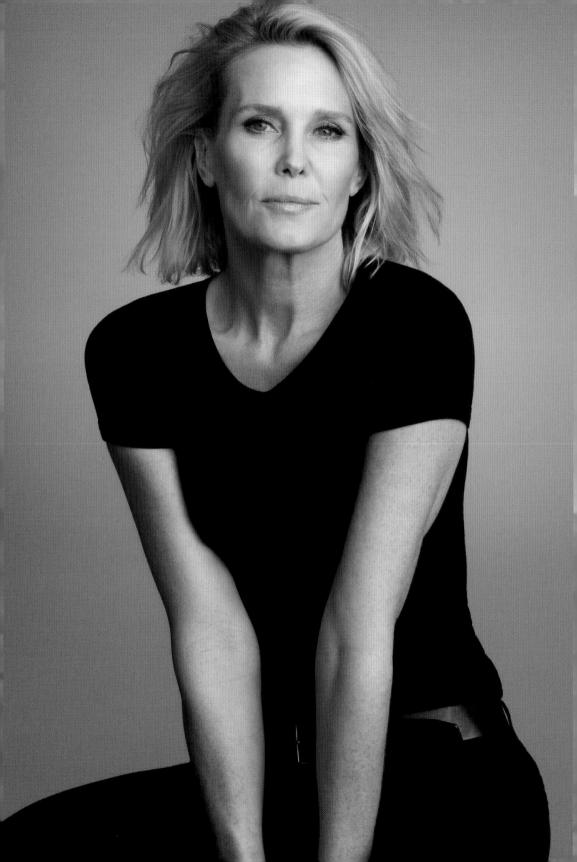

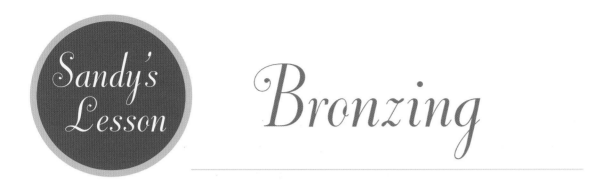

Sandy's Lesson

Bronzing

Nearly every woman has a bronzing powder lurking in her makeup kit. Some women have been wearing it daily for years.

1 **Apply a golden apricot cream highlighter like NARS Orgasm Illuminator to your cheekbone before applying bronzer.** It's my secret to melting the bronzer into your own skin tone.

2 **Choose a bronzing powder compatible in depth of color with your real skin tone.** Be careful not to use a bronzing powder that is too dark for your body skin tone. Face, neck, and décolleté need to match.

3 **Apply bronzing powder with a huge soft bronzing brush for the most believable, even color.** A very full brush picks up, disperses, and sheers the color to prevent a streaky or blotchy look. And here's a reminder to let your under layers of moisturizer and foundation dry completely before applying bronzer, too. I also think everyone knows by now that no matter how terrific or expensive your bronzer, the brush that comes in the compact is totally useless.

4 **Sweep color on your cheekbones and up to the forehead in a C-shape.** This is where the sun hits your bone structure and looks most flattering.

5 **Brush some bronzer on your chin and down the neck for continuity.** You want the bronzer to blend away without obvious borders, especially when you're wearing V necks. Never run bronzer down the center of your nose (which is the most common mistake women make). It gives you a big reddish nose. Instead, use it on the sides of the nose to keep an allover radiance.

6 **Add the lightest touch of cream blush high on the cheekbone.** This is what gives bronzing powder an authentic look and you a glow.

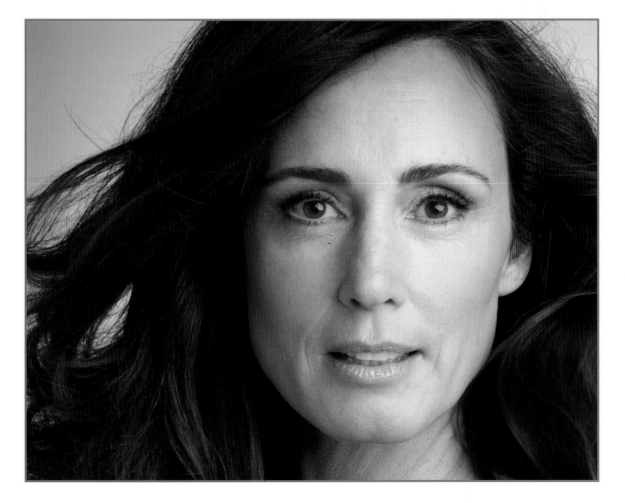

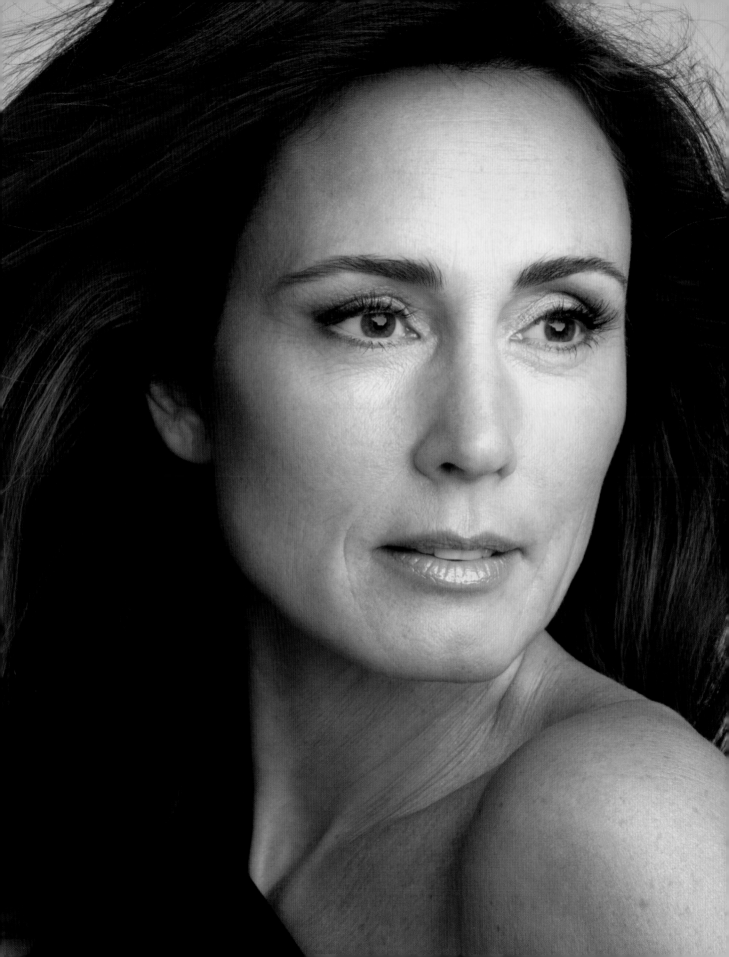

Julie Wolfe

"I'm comfortable with myself now at forty-seven and more confident than I was in my twenties, when I was modeling all over the world. At that time I was one of the few brunettes in the business and I had short hair and a voluptuous figure. Designers like Valentino and Giorgio Armani made giant elastic bras to squash my chest down or strapped my boobs down with ace bandages so I could wear the tiny samples made for flat-chested girls. Once, Armani asked me to lose seven pounds in a week for a job—I suppose they thought my breasts would be the first place I'd lose.

I like my hair long now and I wear little makeup—just tinted moisturizer and mascara. My thick brows were always a trademark and I've been lucky never to fool around with them, so they've stayed in good shape. I was also known for doing lots of swimsuit shoots and I still do them. It's funny, but magazines and advertisers used to send me on location to shoot, and the first few days they always wanted you to work on getting a tan for the shots. I was the Ambre Soleil girl in France and now I get skin checks every six months. Self-tanner is the way to go! I always wear sun block or a hat. I rarely put my face in the sun. My grandmother had amazing skin and she told me *never* go into the sun. She would get upset if she saw me with a tan."

Consider self-tanner
a form of body makeup and
be sure it doesn't end abruptly.
Be sure to include your neck, tops
of hands and feet, and backs
of legs and ankles.

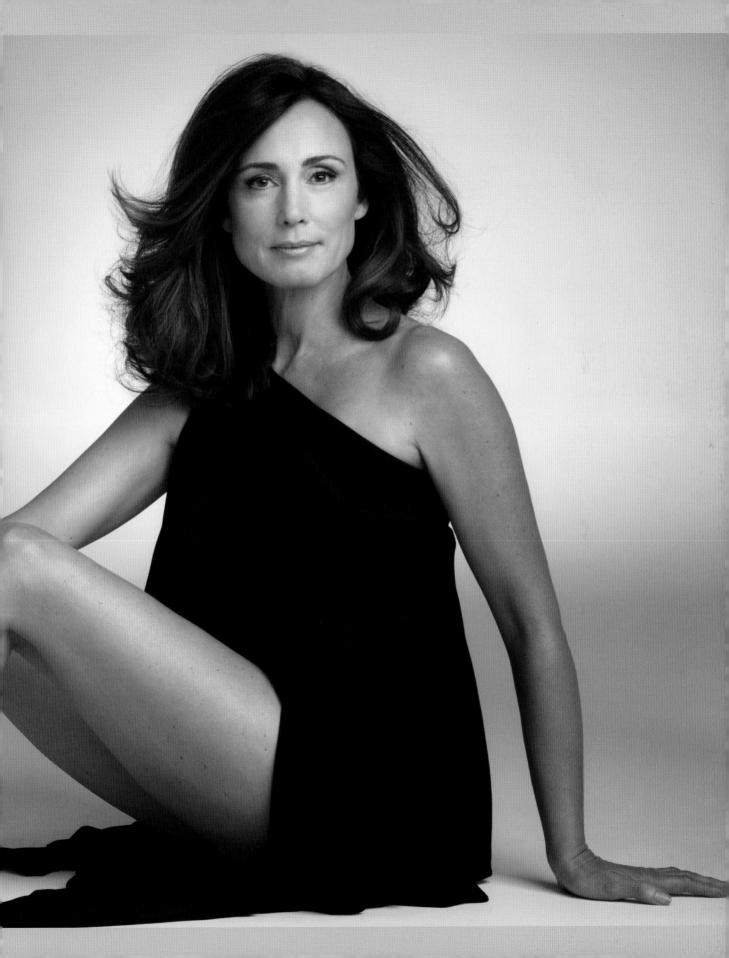

I'm Obsessed with My...

Thin, flat lips: Lip-plumping glosses contain water-retaining ingredients like hyaluronic acid or mild irritants like cinnamon or capsaicin (a chili pepper extract) and can swell your lips slightly for a couple of hours. These aren't dramatic, but temporarily add a little fullness. Light colors with shimmer or shine will enhance thin lips best.

Droopy lips: Make your eyes the real focal point of your makeup. To lift the corners of your mouth though, stick to light, natural lip shades.

Smoker's lines: Diet soda drinkers who used straws for years complain about these grooves above the upper lip too. Dr. Patricia Wexler says the solution is filler: "I inject Restylane into the superficial part of the epidermis perpendicular to the horizontal smoker's lines to smooth them out." Sandy suggests you wear color instead of neutrals on your lips to divert attention away from the lines and that you go for real lipstick instead of gloss.

Dry, creased lips: Prep lips with a lip exfoliating stick to buff off flakes. Then apply a waxy balm (like Chapstick) under your gloss or lipstick to fill in lines. Wear a lipstick or gloss with sunscreen. And stop licking your lips; saliva makes them drier!

Weight gain in the face: Bronzing powder can subtly put back definition and shave away a double chin. Do Sandy's C-shape application to sculpt the cheeks, then blend a small amount of bronzer along the jaw line ear to ear and down the sides of your neck too.

Dull skin: Exfoliate with a polishing scrub or peel before doing your makeup to remove dead skin cells and unclog pores that can give blush a dirty look. Then apply a creamy pink blush to revive a dewy look.

Rosacea/flushed skin: Bronzing powder was made for you. It neutralizes excess redness and turns ruddy, blotchy skin into a healthy vibrant look. Go with it.

Narrow gaunt face: Add fullness to the face with blush high on the cheekbones and follow Sandy's eye and brow elongating tips.

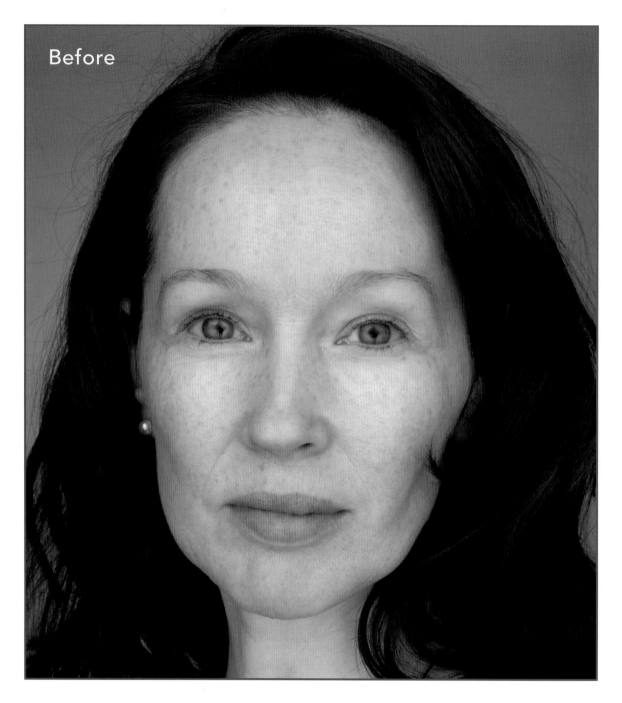

Before

Sun protection works and the proof is seen on Joanne Russell's fair face. Notice how a bright lip color enhances pale skin.

After

blush, bronzer, and lipstick
secrets of celebs and models 40+

Models tweak their signature looks now and then. Even icons like Christie Brinkley, Carol Alt, and Cheryl Tiegs continue to update their signature looks to stay contemporary and relevant. Christie Brinkley emailed us her favorite new trick: a pop of cream blush over her bronzer to make her sunny beach look more realistic and add a glow.

They know extreme dark and light cheek contouring works only on camera. Models who grew up being dramatically sculpted with blush, dark contour powder, and highlighter for photos know it's not for real life.

Celebs adapt color trends but don't copy them. If magazines and the runways are pushing metallic cheek color or bright coral lipstick, celebs and models edit the trends to a texture and color that hints at the news. They might translate the metallic blush to a more wearable shimmery blush, or the coral lip as a peachy gloss, for example.

Models are super picky about lip liner color. You have to find your own neutral. Camera-savvy women know the best shade lip liner matches your own real lip color and it's not "a one size fits all" situation. This is why cosmetic companies have extended their range of lip-toned naturals to include every possible lip shade. If you go too light your lips vanish.

The Top Blush, Bronzer, and Lipstick

Mistakes Most Women Make

Wearing dark lip liner. We don't care if it is a "neutral"! Brown or plum lip pencil gives you ring around the mouth. It's the biggest facial faux pas and it looks tacky. You're not emphasizing or enlarging lip size either this way (if that's your goal); you're shrinking them.

Blending blush into the hairline. Carrying your blush straight up and into your hairline is an old application technique that ended in the '80s. If your hairline has receded or thinned, this is the last place you want to call attention to.

Matching blush to lip color. This is like matching your shoes and bag or fingernails and toes. Why do it? You can have a cool lip and warm cheek or vice versa.

Applying liquid lipstick or dark gloppy glosses like butter. Especially for women with under-defined lips, any lip color that is oozy or liquid can look icky and dated. Keep application thin. We can't say it enough—use a light hand and let the texture and color do the work.

Joanne Russell

"I love makeup. I used to wear it every day but since I had my daughter, Josephine, I don't wear makeup as often as I used to. My mum and brother are always after me to wear more. In the evening I wear dark, heavy eye makeup and a more natural lip. I still like lipstick, though the shades I choose are not as red now. I love stains, especially the ones by CoverGirl, Benefit, and Stila, and if I do nothing else I'll wear one of those. My skin has a tendency to go ruddy, so I wear Revlon ColorStay Mineral Foundation from the drugstore. So far as skincare goes, **I never understood why, as a model in my twenties, I was booked by cosmetic companies for wrinkle cream ads.** Now that I'm forty-eight I realize my English skin, which tends to burn and not tan, saved me from sun damage. I stayed out of the sun because of it; I probably wouldn't have if I'd had the kind of skin that tanned."

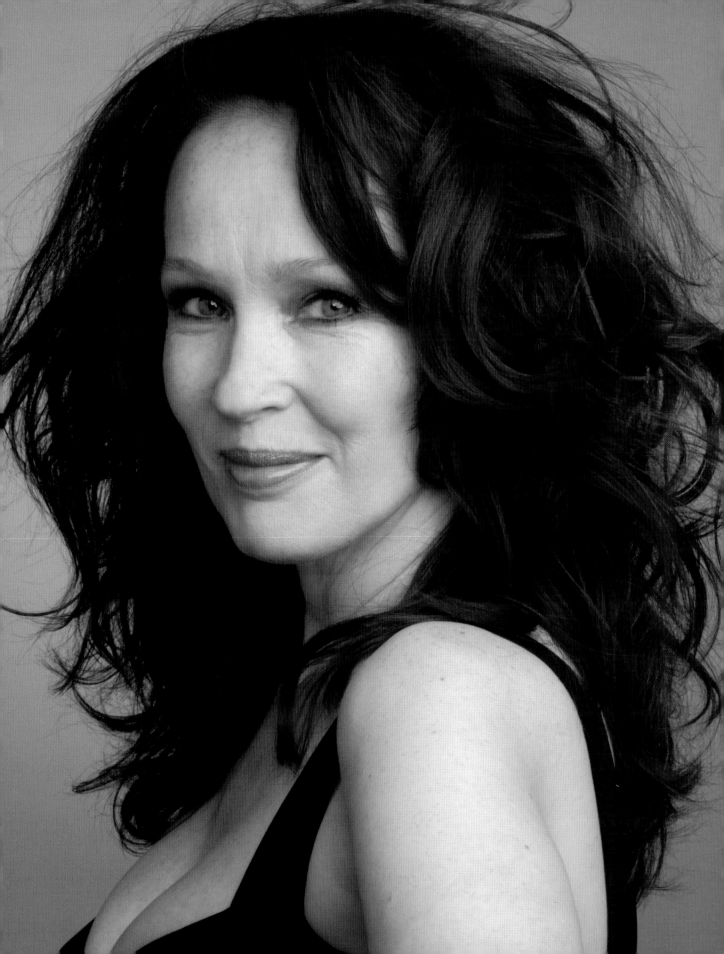

PROS+CONS

As usual, we each have our own blush and lip favorites due to personal preference and our experiences as beauty pros. Sandy's face is more contoured and her lips are well-shaped. I have a narrow, oval face and thin lips. Here's where we differ and why.

Q: **Blush. Cream or powder?**
Shimmer or not?

Women underestimate the value of cheek color. I love blush for its instant ability to make skin look warm and healthy. Even a face cream takes weeks before you see real change. Blush is immediate. There are no hard and fast rules, but blush that's too dark in color will never brighten your skin or add a glow. Blush that's too metallic or glittery just highlights pores and wrinkles. Sheer shimmery blushes work on everyone.

I'm a blush snob. When you have a lot of coverage issues, putting color back into the face after covering all your excess pigment flaws can be tricky. Certain brands get the texture and colors exactly right. These are the ones that turn up in nearly every makeup artist's kit on set and they're the ones I find work best too. Two examples are NARS Orgasm powder blush and Kevyn Aucoin cream blush in Tansoleil or Pravella. They work for absolutely everyone.

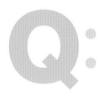

Q: Lips— lipstick or gloss?

Sandy says:

I change my lip color according to my mood. I can wear a deep neutral and switch to a rose gloss an hour later. I personally find gloss worn over lip pencil looks more youthful than lipstick. Whether you choose a real lipstick or gloss absolutely depends on your lips, your personal style, and the moment.

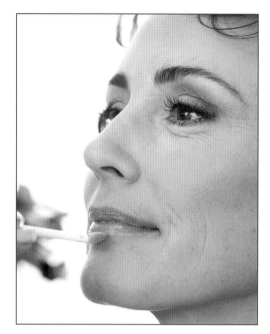

The dark or overly glossy reds we often see in fashion photos on young models are hard to wear and can look messy unless you apply them in thin layers with a brush and have enough shape or volume to handle the intensity. The new high pigment moisturizing lipsticks have increased depth of color and cling without feeling old-fashioned or tacky. If you love color, go for the Lancôme L'Absolu Rouge and Lancôme Le Rouge Absolu lipsticks. Chubby lip pencils are a really great and easy way to use color—especially for women with thin lips because you don't need a lip brush for accuracy.

Lois says:

Because I have small, thin lips I prefer sheer lipsticks, stains, or gloss to full strength lipsticks. Nudes and beiges used to be the only colors I'd wear but I've transitioned into high-pigment sheer lipsticks. They don't look greasy or thick and are easy to wear. So now I do get to wear pinks, roses, and even red. In winter I switch to a rosy berry or a red-tinted balm to treat seasonal dry, cracked lips (a huge problem for me from November to April). And FYI, I'm totally happy with my skinny little lips and have no interest in changing their size with fillers or plumpers! I wish more women would just get over it too.

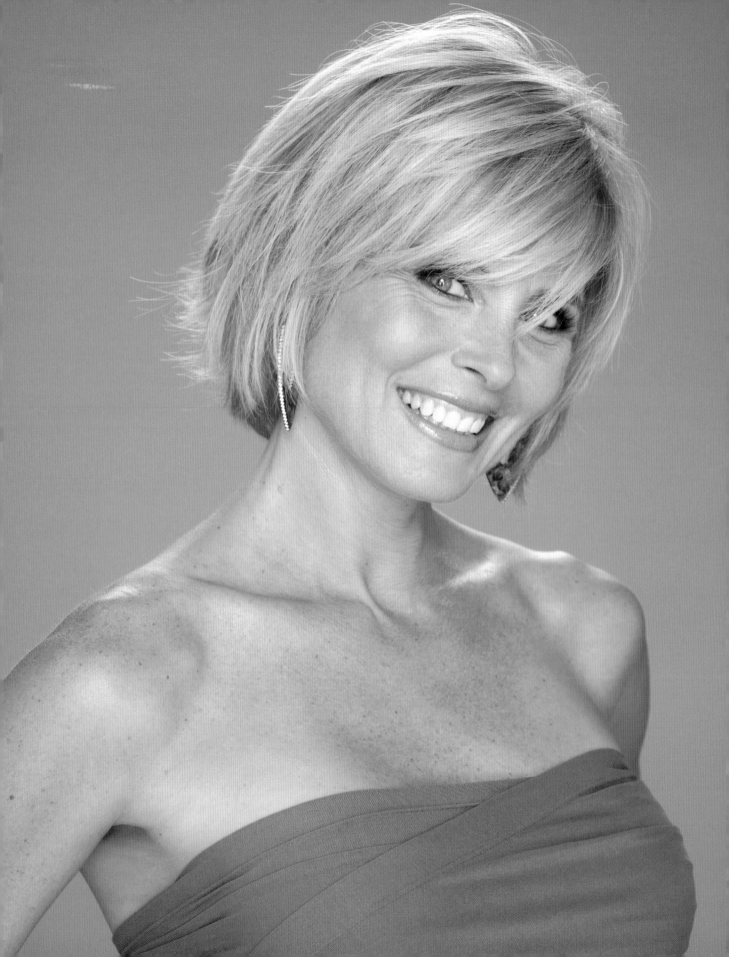

Q : Bronzer. Loose powder or pressed compact?
: Matte or shimmery?

 Sandy says: I prefer powder bronzer in a compact for everyday wear and I believe all bronzers should have shimmer. The only time I use a matte bronzer is when I'm making up a man or a woman with very oily skin.

 Lois says: Bronzing powder is amazing when you're looking fatigued or stressed. My goal is to look like I've actually spent time outdoors, not in front of a computer screen ten hours a day. Sheer bronzers in subtle shades and those with a combination of pink/peach/gold/bronze pigments are easy to wear and don't come off as blatantly fake or overdone.

An extra tip—using a gradual self-tanner early in the morning provides a slight tint neck to toes that makes bronzing powder on the face look real. I love this as an emergency solution!

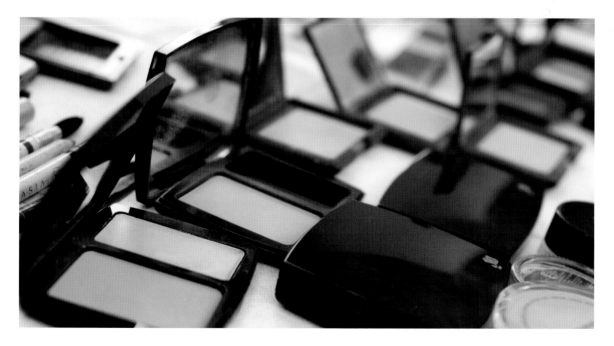

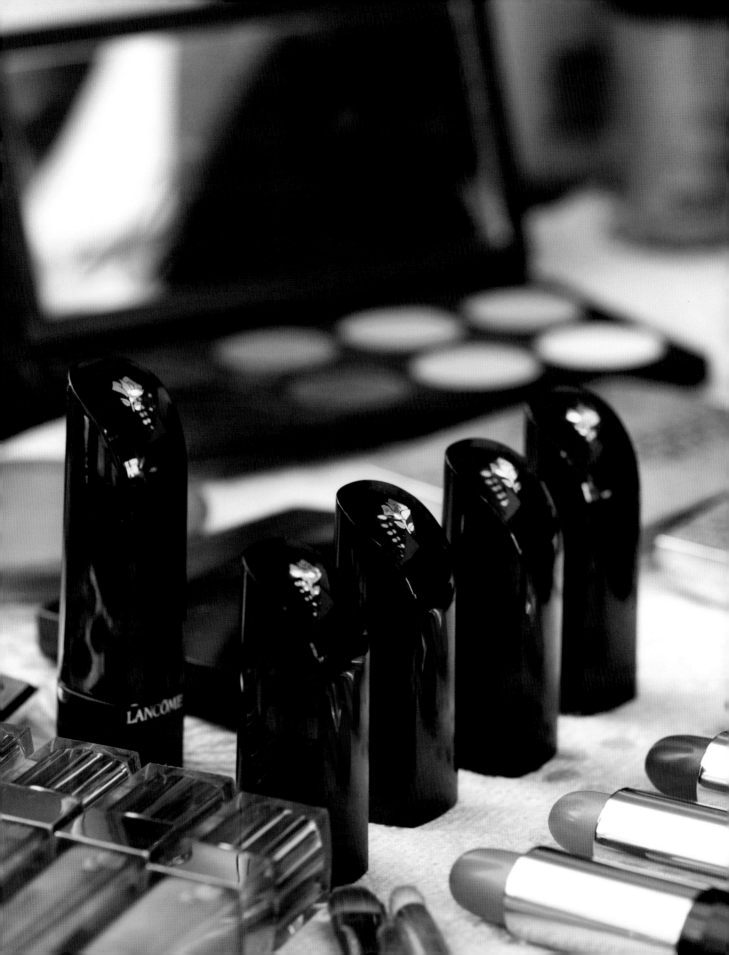

EXPERIENCE

- **Layer gloss over a lip pencil** to achieve more depth of color on thin lips without a heavy lipstick feel.

- **If you're in a tooth whitening mode,** try rose-red or berry lips again.

- **Lips have no defense against UV rays and are a vulnerable spot for skin cancers.** Wear lip protectors with a high SPF or lipsticks with SPF 15 when spending extensive time outdoors.

- **If you're into brights, go for the lip and keep blush subdued.** You can't have equal intensity in both areas, so choose one or the other.

- **If you can splurge on one luxury lipstick, go for a color you'll wear a lot.** Base your splurge selection on need, not crave. Get your color craving out of your system with an inexpensive product.

- **Stains or lip pencils deposit intense pigment with no lipsticky feel.** They are ideal for lipstick haters who dislike any kind of makeup texture.

Lana Ogilvie

"I've been modeling for twenty-two years now and still love it. I used to have a chubby, baby-looking face, but now my bone structure has come through and I have a more chiseled look. I don't like products with fragrance and avoid them, as well as metallics—my skin and eyes are sensitive. Pears soap, Vaseline or Eight Hour Cream on my lips, and Weleda products from the health food store, are my essentials. I've been using organic brands for eighteen years. When I have a casting or I'm going out, I wear mascara (usually L'Oréal), concealer, and maybe a little blush. That's it."

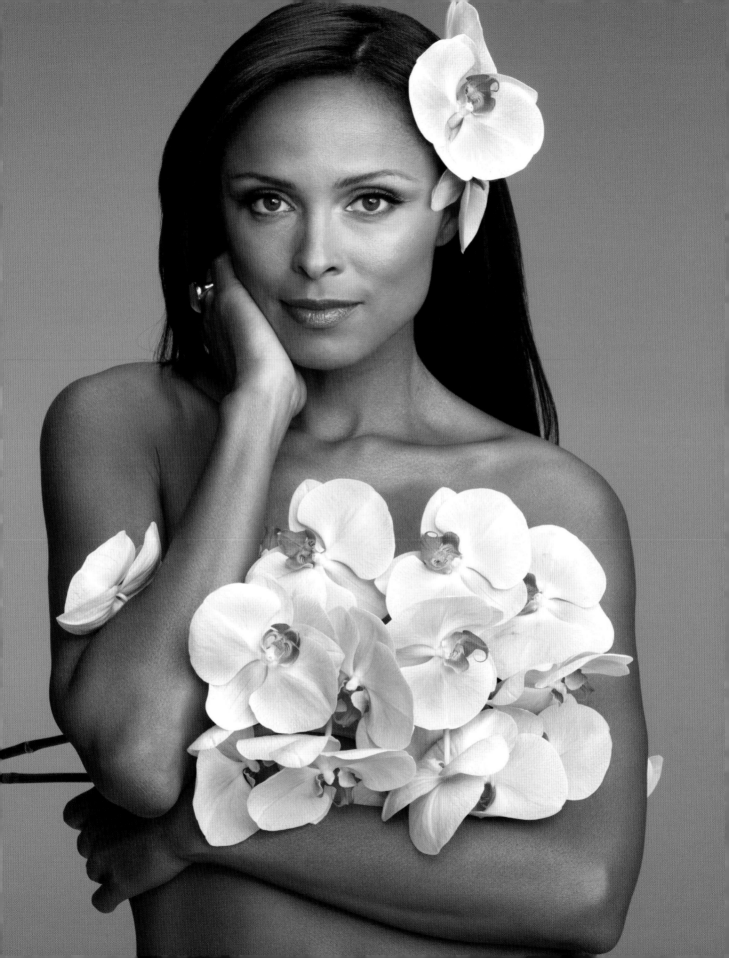

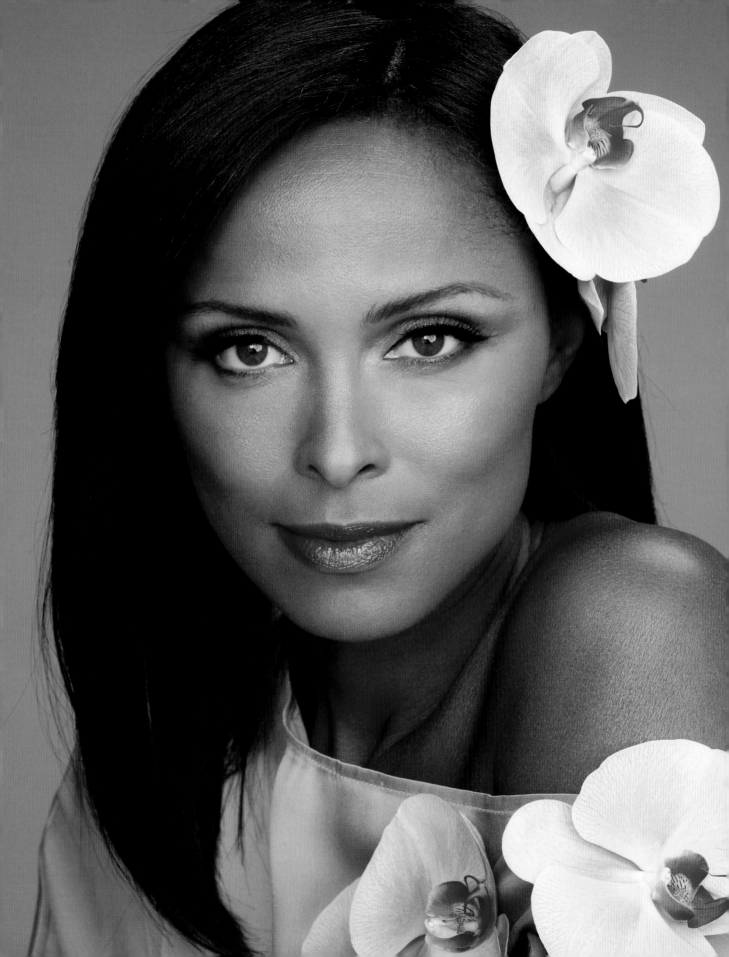

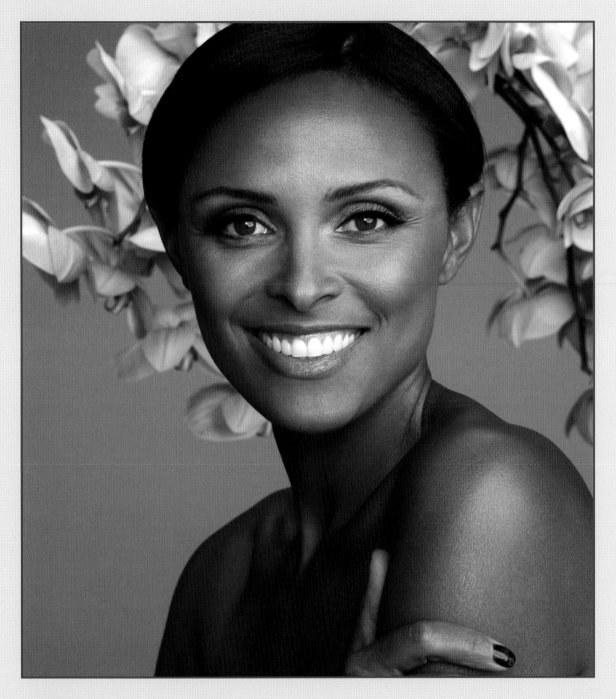

Go for glow on the cheek or the lips— not necessarily both.

The beauty stalkers

Blush

Cream blush:

- **Bobbi Brown Sheer Color Cheek Tint, in Sheer Pink, Sheer Coral, Sheer Raspberry** ($22 bobbibrowncosmetics.com)

- **CoverGirl & Olay Simply Ageless Sculpting Blush, in Plush Peach, Lush Berry** ($10.49 drugstores)

- **Giorgio Armani Blushing Fabric, in Pink Chiffon, Shimmering Peach, Sicilian Orange** ($38 giorgioarmanibeauty-usa.com)

- **Kevyn Aucoin The Creamy Moist Glow, in Tansoleil, Pravella, Bliss, Euphoria** ($24 kevynaucoin.com)

- **M.A.C. Blushcreme, in Posey, Ladyblush, Lilicent, Laid Back** ($18.50 maccosmetics.com)

- **NARS Cream Blush, in Guele de Nuit, Penny Lane, Constantinople, Turkish Red** ($26 narscosmetics.com)

- **Stila Convertible Color, in Gerbera, Petunia, Rose, Lillium** ($25 stilacosmetics.com)

Powder blush:

- **Bobbi Brown Shimmer Blush, in Pink Sugar, Pink Coral, Washed Rose** ($22 bobbibrowncosmetics.com)

- **Lancôme Blush Subtil, in Evening After, Pink L'Amour, Rose Fresque, Rose Romantique** ($29.50 lancome-usa.com)

- **M.A.C. Powder Blush, in Instant Chic, Pink Swoon, Tenderling, Peach Twist, Sincere, Springsheen** ($18.50 maccosmetics.com)

- **Kevyn Aucoin The Pure Powder Glow, in Shadore, Myracle, Fira, and Dolline** ($37 kevynaucoin.com)

go shopping for

- **NARS Powder Blush, in Orgasm, Amour, Desire, Dolce Vita, Mata Hari** ($26 narscosmetics.com)

Bronzer

- **Bobbi Brown Illuminating Bronzing Powder** ($33 bobbibrowncosmetics.com)
- **Laura Mercier Bronzing Duo** ($32 lauramercier.com)
- **L'Oréal Paris Glam Bronze Bronzing Powder** ($12.99 drugstores)
- **Edward Bess Ultra Luminous Bronzer** ($48 bergdorfgoodman.com)
- **Guerlain Terracotta Bronzing Powder** ($47 sephora.com)
- **Lancôme Star Bronzer Sun-Kissed Bronzing Powder** ($36.50 lancome-usa.com)
- **Revlon Beyond Natural Blush & Bronzer** ($11 drugstores)
- **Yves Saint Laurent Bronzing Powder** ($48 yslbeautyus.com)

Highlighter

- **NARS Orgasm Illuminator** ($29 sephora.com)

Serious lip treatments

Great overnight or home-alone healers for chapped lips:

- **Elizabeth Arden Eight Hour Cream Skin Protectant** ($17 elizabetharden.com)
- **Aquaphor Healing Ointment** ($5.09 drugstores)

- **Kiehl's Since 1851 Lip Balm, #1** ($7 kiehls.com)
- **La Mer The Lip Balm** ($45 cremedelamer.com)

Tinted lip balms

For dry, cracked, flaky lips:

- **Bobbi Brown Tinted Lip Balm** ($18 bobbibrowncosmetics.com)
- **Dior Crème de Rose Lip Balm** ($25 sephora.com)
- **Fresh Sugar Rose Tinted Lip Treatment** ($22.50 sephora.com)
- **Laura Mercier Hydratint Lip Balm SPF 15** ($20 lauramercier.com)

High-pigment, hydrating lipsticks

For great texture and modern color:

- **Bobbi Brown Lip Color, in Brownie Pink, Slopes, Rose, Rose Berry** ($22 bobbibrowncosmetics.com)
- **Chanel Rouge Allure Luminous Satin Lip Colour, in Desirable, Comedia, Attitude, Lover, Libertine** ($30 chanel.com)
- **Clinique High Impact Lip Color SPF 15, in Citrus Rose, Red-y to Wear, Extreme Pink, Nude Beach, Rosette** ($14 clinique.com)
- **Estée Lauder Signature Hydra Lustre Lipstick, in Cinnamon, Chelsea Rose, Lustrous Pink** ($19.50 esteelauder.com)
- **Giorgio Armani Rouge d'Armani Lipstick, #103, #503, #506, #507, #508** ($30 giorgioarmanibeauty-usa.com)
- **Lancôme L'Absolu Rouge, in Absolute Rouge, Fleur de Lis, Champagne, Coquette, Blush Classique, Berry Noir** ($29 lancome-usa.com)
- **Laura Mercier Creme Lip Colour, in Audrey, Caramel, Cinnamon, Dry Rose** ($22 lauramercier.com)
- **Maybelline Color Sensational Lipcolor, in Born With It, Pinkalicious, Plaza Pink, Warm Me Up, Tinted Taupe** ($7.49 drugstores)

- Yves Saint Laurent Rouge Volupté Silky Sensual Radiant Lipstick SPF 15, in Lingerie Pink, Provocative Pink, Red Muse, Rose Paris, Faubourg Peach ($34 yslbeautyus.com)

Sheer color lipsticks in natural or pow-y shades:

- Laura Mercier Sheer Lip Colour, in Sexy Lips, Tender Lips, Healthy Lips, Baby Lips ($20 lauramercier.com)
- Shiseido Makeup Perfect Sheer Lip Color, in Tender PK327, Natural Red RD629, Pout RS326 ($25 nordstrom.com)
- Trish McEvoy Sheer Lip Color, in Jolie, Sheer Milan, Sheer London ($23 nordstrom.com)
- Yves Saint Laurent Rouge Pur Shine Sheer Lipstick SPF 15, in Natural Pink, Brick Red ($30 yslbeautyus.com)

Lip glosses

For perfect non-tacky shine:

- Bobbi Brown Brightening Lip Gloss, in ANY shade! ($20 bobbibrowncosmetics.com)
- Chanel Glossimer, in Magnifique, Courtisane ($27 chanel.com)
- Clé de Peau Beauté Lip Gloss, in N3, N5, N10, N11 ($48 neimanmarcus.com)
- Lancôme Color Fever Lip Gloss Sensual Vibrant Lip Shine, in Mercury Rising, Blazing Pink ($26 lancome-usa.com)
- Maybelline Color Sensational Lip Gloss, in Born With It, Pink Perfection, Sugared Honey, Mocha Glaze ($6.49 drugstores)
- Trish McEvoy Beauty Booster Lip Gloss SPF 15, in Very Sexy, Sexy Rose, Sexy Peach ($25 nordstrom.com)
- Yves Saint Laurent Golden Gloss Shimmering Lip Gloss, in Golden Pink, Golden Petal, Golden Praline ($30 yslbeautyus.com)

For creamy gloss with denser, lipstick-like coverage:

- Bobbi Brown Lip Gloss, in Rosey, Pink Beige, Petal ($20 bobbibrowncosmetics.com)

- Estée Lauder Pure Color Gloss Stick, in Honey Pink, Berry Pink, Nude Almond ($20 esteelauder.com)

- Lancôme L'Absolu Crème de Brilliance, in Rose Mystique, Exotic Orchid, Sienna Ultime, Champagne ($29 lancome-usa.com)

- Lancôme La Laque Fever Lipshine, in Lucent Nude, Feverish, Plum Wave ($26 lancome-usa.com)

- M.A.C. Cremesheen Glass, in Just Superb, Deelight, Over Indulgence ($18 maccosmetics.com)

Lip stains

For stay-there color and precision:

- CoverGirl Outlast Lipstain, in Wild Berry Wink, Berry Smooch ($7.29 drugstores)
- Laura Mercier Lip Stain, in English Rose, Scarlet, Hibiscus ($20 sephora.com)

Lip liners

To correct asymmetries:

- Bobbi Brown Lip Liner ($22 bobbibrowncosmetics.com)
- Kevyn Aucoin Lip Liner ($24 kevynaucoin.com)
- Lancôme Le Crayon Lip Contour ($22.50 lancome-usa.com)
- NARS Lip Liner ($18.50 sephora.com)

Chubby lip pencils

To correct and fill in with a creamy finish:

- Bobbi Brown Lip Crayon, in Honeysuckle, Posey, Wild Rose, Raisin Berry ($22 bobbibrowncosmetics.com)

- NARS Velvet Matte Pencil, in Dolce Vita, Belle de Jour, Bettina ($24 sephora.com)

- Shiseido Makeup Automatic Lip Crayon, in Lc6, Lc4 ($23 nordstrom.com)
- Sonia Kashuk for Target Lip Crayon, in Berry Nude, Pinky Nude, Nudey Nude

  ($7.99 target.com)
- Trish McEvoy Essential Pencil, in Model's Choice, Baby Pink, Nude

  ($25 saksfifthavenue.com)

Blush, bronzer, and lip brushes

Lip brushes:

- NARS Retractable Lip Brush, #11 ($26 narscosmetics.com)
- Giorgio Armani Lip Brush ($25 giorgioarmanibeauty-usa.com)
- Laura Mercier Lip Colour Brush ($24 lauramercier.com)
- Shu Uemura Natural Brush, 6m ($24 shuuemura-usa.com)

Blush brushes:

- Chanel Blush Brush, #7 ($46 chanel.com)
- Lancôme Precision Cheek Brush, #7 ($47.50 lancome-usa.com)
- Laura Mercier Cheek Colour Brush ($45 lauramercier.com)
- Laura Mercier Crème Cheek Color Brush ($36 lauramercier.com)

Cream blush brushes:

- Shu Uemura Natural Brush, #17, #20 ($50 shuuemura-usa.com)
- Shu Uemura Synthetic Brush, #14 ($40 shuuemura-usa.com)

Bronzer brushes:

- M.A.C. Powder/Blush Brush ($34 maccosmetics.com)
- Bobbi Brown Bronzer Brush ($50 bobbibrowncosmetics.com)
- Giorgio Armani Blush Brush ($44 saksfifthavenue.com)
- NARS Bronzing Brush ($52 narscosmetics.com)

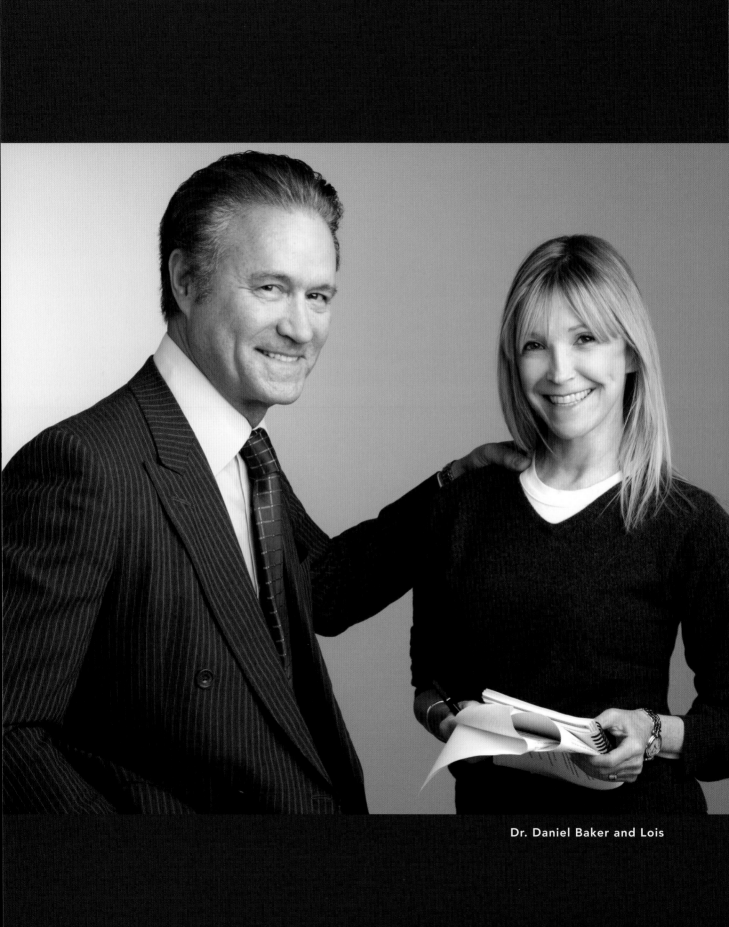

Dr. Daniel Baker and Lois

CHAPTER FIVE

Should I Get Some Work Done?

Yes? No? Maybe?

Lois + Sandy Solve the Dilemma (with help from a few M.D.s)

What woman doesn't look in the mirror, pull back her skin for a crease-free face, and glimpse a possible facelift? We all do—even those of us who talk about "aging gracefully."

Vanity is a toughie for women living in our youth-oriented, celebrity-obsessed culture, where TV anchors moan about the revelations of pores and lines on HDTV. We know gorgeous women at forty-eight who live in turtlenecks, scarves, and sunglasses to hide their necks, jaw lines, and under-eye bags (even in the heat of Miami and Phoenix!). We've met fabulous-looking women at fifty who won't cut their shoulder length hair or pull it back because their "jowls" will show. There are amazing women at fifty-five who insist on heavy, dated foundation and concealer to hide their brown spots and circles. We know sexy babes of sixty who have given up on liner and shadow because their eyes are so deep-set or baggy. Sandy says the best makeup in the world isn't going to do enough if you truly believe your issues are beyond cosmetic control. Never do plastic surgery to please anyone but you. Only you can decide how far to go when it comes to your looks.

Let's be realistic. Everyone knows celebrities, politicians, corporate execs, newsmakers, and big-name models "do things" to refresh their appearance. If your face was twenty-feet high on a movie screen, if you needed to look great on TV, if you were using media visibility to grow your brand, or you were constantly snapped by paparazzi, you would too. A very famous blonde sixty-ish actress once told Lois regarding makeup, "You need to do less the older you get—that's the secret." Lois says, "I actually believed her until I found out the 'less' was one fabulous facelift instead of twenty products."

Some women are, as the French used to say, "comfortable in your own skin" and can easily ignore the whole cosmetic surgery/Botox world of procedures and treatments. Makeup, great

> Looks are part of the package that includes knowledge, experience, and confidence—things that make women comfortable with the aging process.

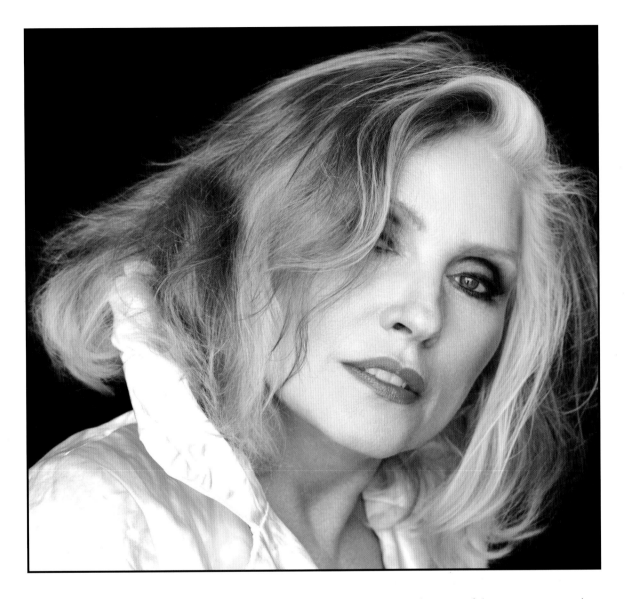

hair color, a contemporary haircut, and stylish clothes are all they need. Many of these women say they don't want to become cosmetic surgery junkies or look "done."

But there are other women who want to enhance their looks when makeup alone doesn't offer them enough of a change. The democratization of cosmetic surgery (thanks to reality TV and the Internet) has made it more available and accessible than ever before. Surgery or dermatological procedures alone won't provide the solution though; they need to work hand-in-hand with makeup to maximize the benefits.

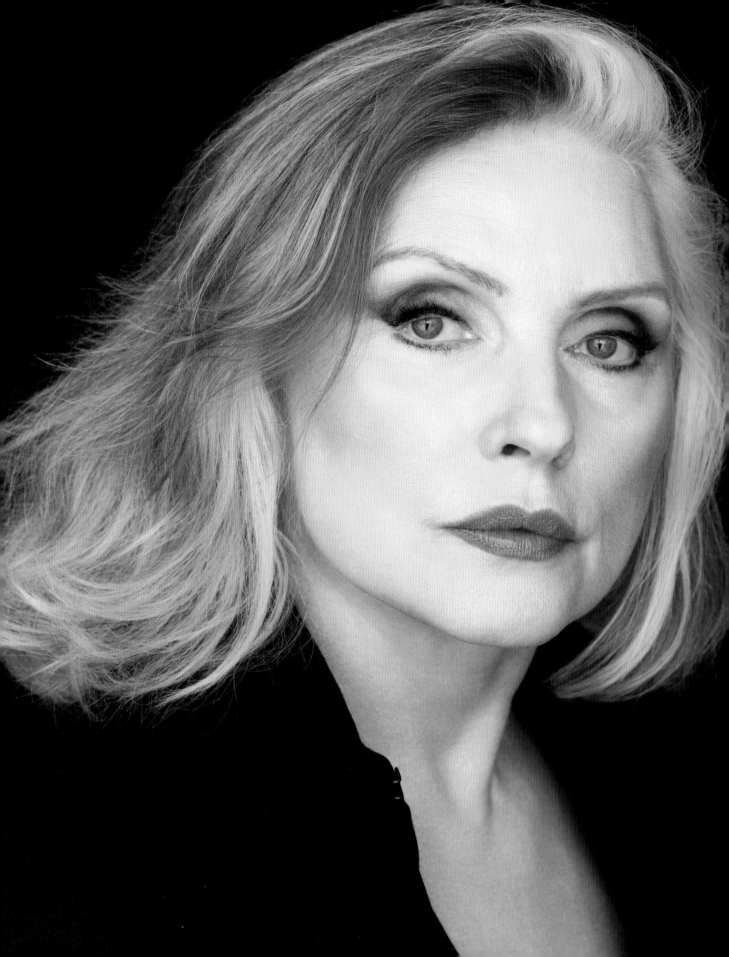

Deborah Harry

"I feel pretty good about being sixty-five. As women, we're never objective about our look; we're microscopic. This is true whether or not you make your living from your looks and are in the public eye. I've had very good cosmetic surgery—a facelift by Dr. Dan Baker ten years ago and it still looks great. My feeling is if it makes you happy, do it! The thing that bothers me the most now are my brows—they're unmanageable, wiry, and coarse, like a fisherman sitting in a dinghy on the North Sea somewhere. They're the worst! They require lots of work trimming, grooming, shaping, but I really can't complain. I'm a very lucky girl."

We asked a team of top medical experts for their take on procedures and practices. Meet:

Dr. Daniel Baker, superstar New York City cosmetic surgeon to celebrities, socialites, A-list fashion designers, supermodels, and beauty-industry honchos.

Dr. Fredric Brandt, Botox and filler guru to models, rock stars, and fashion designers with offices in New York City and Coral Gables, Florida.

Dr. Patricia Wexler, NYC star cosmetic dermatologist with a hush-hush clientele of beauty editors, actors, and fashion designers.

Here's how this chapter works:

For each procedure or situation our experts offer their insights and advice, and then we put in our two cents. If you pass and decide to solve the issue without medical intervention at this time, Sandy and I give you a beauty solution.

The Facelift

It's the ultimate leap. Yes, it means cutting, stitching, and a recovery time of two weeks, but what you buy is a do-over and freedom from thinking about saggy skin at the jaw and neck for at least ten to twelve years.

10 Crucial Tips to Know Before You Get a Facelift: A private consultation with Dr. Daniel Baker

Dr. Baker's schedule is booked so far in advance (as are most top surgeons) that even movie stars schedule their filming around his calendar. He's also one of the most down-to-earth, honest guys we know, so who better to ask?

1 **A facelift will get you back to where you were.** "I'm not Michelangelo. I'm an artisan and I have an aesthetic sensibility, but I don't try to transform people into something they're not. Women see movie stars in magazines, on TV, or in films, and think they always look that way. If you saw them in person you might be surprised. Makeup pros, lighting, and Photoshop change and enhance most magazine photos."

2 **The patient needs to take responsibility too.** "Facelift surgery is a personal investment which you control and manage by maintaining a stable body weight, diet, exercise, and sun protection. Consider the cost, the recovery time, and the fact that you want results to last as long as possible. Getting in the best possible shape before surgery is a smart idea. You need to stop smoking because smoking delays healing. New fat, and by that I mean recent weight gain, needs to go. You can reverse it with diet and exercise."

3 **Do a lift sooner rather than later.** "I feel strongly about doing your first facelift when it will give you the greatest amount of pleasure from the results and that's probably going to be in your mid- to late-forties—this is prime time for most women. Then maybe you might add a few little tweaks to extend the result. This is when you're socially active, have a career, have finished having kids, you're in good shape, maybe dating or

in a relationship, and in good health, so why not enjoy the benefits early? It's more about maintenance than starting over and it will keep you looking your best for ten to twelve years."

4 The modern facelift is not just about tightening. "It's also about restoring volume, often with your own fat; resurfacing the skin with a peel; and doing Botox all at once. It's a much more pragmatic approach than it was before. A facelift alone—firming up the neck and jowls—will make a major, 95 percent improvement in your looks. Every face is different and there are limitations. Adding filler or fat or doing some resurfacing may be necessary to get the maximum result and I usually address this accordingly at the time of surgery. I call it 'The Rejuvenation Facelift.' There's one anesthesia, one recovery and downtime, one period of bruising, so it's more efficient.

The first thing I ask patients is, 'What bothers you?' It's important to address your concerns in the consultation, because a good surgeon will not suggest making additional changes unless you bring them up. If you're unhappy with your nose or eyes too, it's your responsibility as a patient to discuss this with your doctor when you talk about your facelift because a good surgeon won't bring it up otherwise. Think carefully about what you want to achieve and improve and participate in the evaluation. It's best not to change things that do not bother you—doing too much is what makes you look unnatural."

5 A good facelift should last 10 to 12 years. "Usually if I do someone at fifty, they'll come again at sixty. I have patients who have had three facelifts, one every ten years. They're active, energetic women who are working and want to make the most of their looks. If the surgery is done correctly, a redone facelift will still look natural."

6 Get a lift when you're feeling up, not down. "Surgery cannot change the involuntary expression of the face. A surgeon needs to be careful about the emotional stability of patients. A recent widow, someone who is in a depression, may be

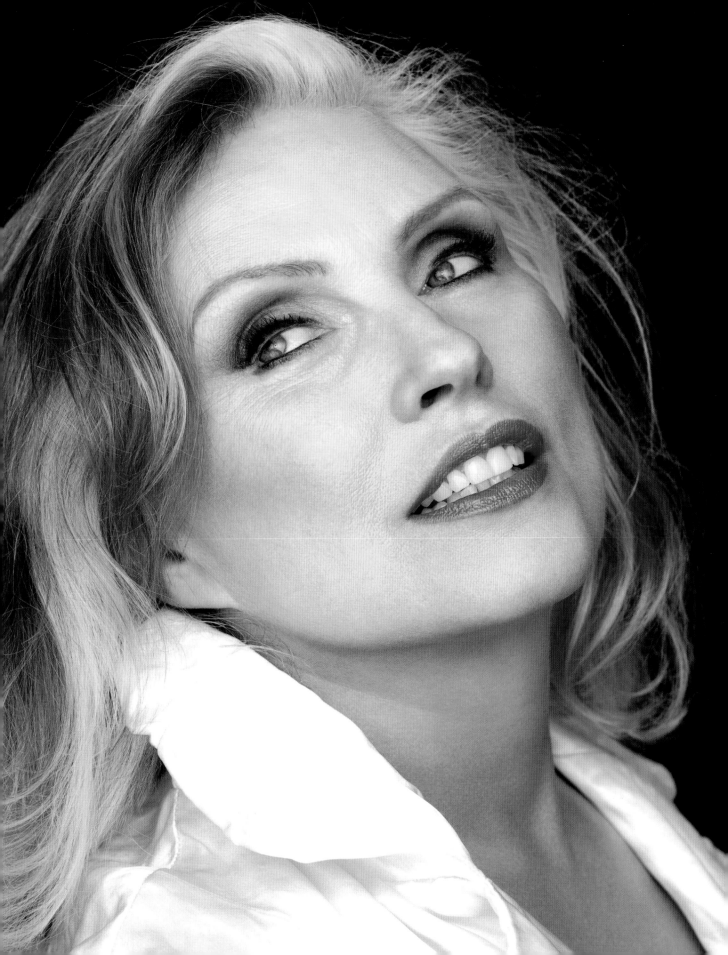

wise to put off surgery for a while and resolve issues. Wait until you're rested and in a better place emotionally to appreciate the results of a facelift. This is something special you are doing for yourself and you need to be in the best emotional and physical shape."

7 The surgeon's aesthetic judgment makes the difference.

"How the skin is redraped, how much fat is removed or added, and how the face is sculpted makes all the difference—not the type of lift. Facelift techniques are always being modified and improved, so lifts done ten years ago have been revised even when the basic procedures remain the same. All surgeons have technical abilities; the main difference is the surgeon's aesthetic judgment. There are no secrets or 'best' facelift techniques.

One of the biggest problems I see now is women who have done too much to their lips. The overdone lip—the big lip filler trend—is just out of control. Some women have even had permanent lip fillers inserted (and badly); the only thing you can do is cut them out. When a new patient comes in wanting her face done and she has already done way too much filler to her lips and face, I say forget it; why don't you skip fillers for a while and come back six months from now to talk."

8 A facelift is cost efficient in the long run.

"If you figure out what you spend over a period of five or six years on fillers, Botox, and dermatological procedures, you could pay for two facelifts! In my opinion, it's not cost effective in the end if you're a high-maintenance type who continuously goes for procedures. I will say, however, that fillers and Botox are excellent additions to certain areas surgery cannot address."

9 "Lunchtime facelifts" claiming no pain, no scars, no downtime, are BS.

"You can get bad surgery anywhere—it's the surgeon, not the procedure. One third of the patients I see have had bad surgery elsewhere; there were complications, the results look weird or obvious, the results didn't last, or they look overdone. Women seeking surgery are customers and they will be sold as much as they can be sold on getting a deal.

Some commercial facelifts are being marketed as mini-lifts on TV in ads and online, claiming to remove wrinkles and saggy skin in an hour with only a local anesthetic. Patients who seek these one-size-fits-all branded quickie nips and tucks are buying procedure, not the surgeon's credentials. A lot of these end up in re-dos, with traditional lifts making up for mini-results."

It's up to you to decide what not to do—and that's actually more important than what you do.

10 The best way to find a doctor is through referrals from other doctors or friends who have had positive experiences.

"Women are now really customers, not patients. There are a lot of tacky websites out there and magazines with best doctor listings that are not reliable. Neither of these sources is a good way to pick a cosmetic surgeon. A lot of surgeons represented are just good salesmen and good marketers rather than reputable surgeons with the right kind of aesthetics. Magazine articles or TV shows are not a good way to select a surgeon either."

SANDY + LOIS *say:*

if you decide to get a facelift . . .

- **It's essential to still look like you.** We've seen women (even celebrities) lose their identity post-surgery because they do too much. Use the words "I want to look natural and fresh" during your consultation.

- **Do the get-healthy part first. Staying healthy and fit should be a goal whether you opt for surgery or stick with makeup.** Smoke? Tan? Skip the sunscreen? Drink alcohol in excess? All of these are bad habits to let go of forever. What you did to your face pre-op determines how quickly you heal. The recovery period after a facelift may include swelling, redness tissue formation (hopefully not!), tightness, and bruising. It's a good idea to get your teeth whitened and have any dental work done a month or so before your surgery.

- **Be patient. Post-surgery recovery is a phase you just have to go through.** Your face and neck may feel tight or numb for months, even up to a year. Some women actually love that feeling of tightness and crave it when it's gone. It does eventually go away. The incisions are wounds that need time to heal completely, even after stitches are out, before you can cover them with makeup. Incision scars start out deep red then fade to pink.

- **There are certain things you will be putting off for quite a while.** We hope we don't have to remind you, but of course skip self-tanner, spray tan booths, facials, face masks, saunas, and at-home microdermabrasion, exfoliation, or peels until you are fully healed.

- **You will want a sunblock of at least SPF 30 to protect the scars from the sun once they have healed,** especially if you do outdoor sports or gardening or live in a sunny climate.

- **Once you heal, you'll find your cheeks have once again moved up and into place.** This will allow you to wear blush once again on the round apples of your cheeks, and play with lip colors that call attention to your lower face.

- **When you are at home recovering from cosmetic surgery be careful around your cats and dogs.** These pets can transmit the drug-resistant germ MRSA to the wound area, resulting in a serious infection. Frequent washing or sanitizing of your hands before and after playing with a pet, or wearing gloves during this time, is a smart precaution. Do not let them lick your face and do not wash pet food or water bowls in the same sink where you prepare food.

- **If you've had your eyes done too, opt for big lightweight sunglasses that won't rest too heavily on your face or the bridge of your nose.** Tom Ford's superlight aviators are incredible for post-surgery.

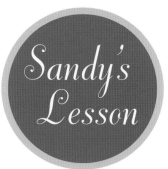

Sandy's Lesson

Post-op Makeup

Q: How do you hide the bruising and get back to work and life?

1 **Buy special camouflage makeup that's creamy, but opaque and water-resistant.** Don't make the mistake of trying to use your usual makeup—there simply isn't enough coverage. Order a skin-tone shade online before your surgery so you have it ready when your surgeon gives the OK. Get the setting powder that is sold with the cover-up, too. It seals the cream and locks it in place. We recommend CM-Beauty by Covermark Classic Cover and CM-Beauty by Covermark Finishing Powder, or Dermablend Cover Creme Foundation SPF 30 and Dermablend Setting Powder. By whatever miracle, these creams melt seamlessly into your skin and won't give dark bruised areas a gray look. They also don't transfer.

Skip camouflage in corrective shades of green, orange, yellow, and lavender that claim to counteract discolorations. You'll look like you're ready for an autopsy!

2 **Be light-handed in applying cover-up to bruised post-surgery areas.** There should be absolutely no rubbing, stretching, or pulling of the skin. The last thing you want is to promote any irritation that will slow the healing process. If you've had serious laser resurfacing along with your lift, your doctor will have prescribed an ointment to keep this area moist while it's healing, so any camouflage makeup will have to wait at the very least ten days. Bruises start out purple and fade to green, then yellow.

This takes at least two weeks so don't be shocked. Please don't think about applying any kind of makeup before your doctor gives the final OK— no matter what your friends say.

3 **Use the back of your hand as a palette and apply your special camouflage with a concealer brush.** Warm a dab of camouflage on the back of your hand. Then, using a gentle patting motion, brush on the concealer cream and continue to pat until all bruises are covered. Feather the edges so they fade right into your skin with no lines of demarcation.

4 **Set the cream with a very light touch of loose powder.** It prevents the camouflage from moving or coming off on your phone.

Thanks, but no facelift for now. What can makeup alone do?

Aim for a polished look (which you'll learn more about in Chapter 6). Emphasize your upper face with defined eye makeup and blush high on the cheekbone. This will help draw attention away from your jaw line and neck. Keep as much attention as possible on your upper face by getting your brows back in shape or cutting bangs.

Refreshing an Old Facelift

After you've had a facelift, your face continues to age. The new "non-surgical facelift"—a combination of less invasive treatments—might be your next move if you decide to skip another lift once the skin begins to sag again.

Dr. Fredric Brandt says: "There are four key things you can do to refresh an old facelift or rejuvenate a sun-damaged face when you don't want cosmetic surgery. One, resurface with laser or peels to improve skin texture. Two, use fillers like Restylane or Perlane to add volume to the face. Three, relax forehead creases and neck cords with Botox. Four, tighten saggy skin with Thermage or laser (although the last is not a home run, like the first three)."

 SANDY +LOIS say: If you're going to spend the time and money to refresh your face with dermatological solutions, don't continue with the same old makeup. It's like losing ten pounds and continuing to dress in baggy, shape-hiding clothes.

Thanks, but no more surgery or dermatological help for now. What can makeup and haircolor alone do?

A lot. Even if you just improve your application technique and use the products you own differently, you've pulled ahead. Makeup won't restore the tight, taut feeling of a facelift but it will give you a fresh shot of confidence and a new look, especially if you update the colors and textures. Update your hair cut and color too. We consulted two celebrity hairstylists in NYC: haircolor guru Brad Johns

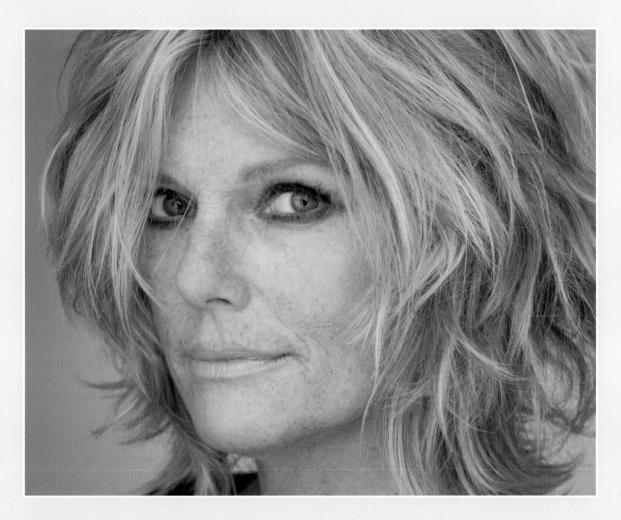

of the Brad Johns Color Studio at the Elizabeth Arden Red Door Salon and beauty trendsetter Rita Hazan of the Rita Hazan Salon.

Brad says: "Work with your looks as an entire package. Avoid extremes like a super-trendy cut or switching from highlights to solid color because either one will emphasize age-related skin issues."

Rita says: "Do some research and splurge once on a consultation with a top colorist. Usually changing color that's too dark, too light, or too red can de-age you in a few hours. Your skin has lost pigment and replacing the warmth in your hair while softening the color makes a huge difference to your overall look. Your own colorist can then maintain the results."

Saggy Neck, Double Chin

We'd love to ignore the little wattle under our chins, the noticeable cords, and the tell-tale rings around our necks. Though it's not the same as a face and necklift, Botox can actually slurp up a small amount of loose skin under the chin and tighten muscle cords and slightly crepey skin.

Dr. Fredric Brandt says: "Botox can do a lot to tighten a saggy neck if a facelift is not on your agenda. Strategic injections into your muscles can relax the platysma muscles in the neck to get rid of cords and rings. You will probably need a few rows of several injections each to accomplish this, but it does work for my patients and lasts up to six months."

SANDY +LOIS say: Look at your face and neck in profile too when you do your makeup and hair. This is how a lot of the world sees you every day. A trick models do to tighten the area under the chin (especially for photos) is to press the flat part of your tongue against the roof of your mouth while you smile. It works. Try it!

Sandy agrees with Dr. Baker: "Injections in my neck would wind up being too costly. I personally opted for a necklift by Dr. David Rosenberg." Lois thinks: "Expanding your skincare and sunscreen to your neck and chest is one of the smartest things you can do—especially after a costly facelift. If I buy a special neck cream for that area I don't neglect to use it."

Thanks, but no surgery for now.
What can makeup and style do?

Work at creating the illusion of a longer, smoother neck. When applying foundation, use a damp sponge to gently buff your base over the "cliff" of the jaw and then down onto the neck. Use a light contour powder to define the jaw line. Use strongly pigmented matte taupe shades for definition. You can also substitute bronzer for contour powder.

Opt for V necklines instead of hiding in turtlenecks. Showing more skin at the throat and upper chest, where the skin is smooth and firm, elongates the appearance of the neck. Don't go too low though— you've gone too far if you're showing cleavage.

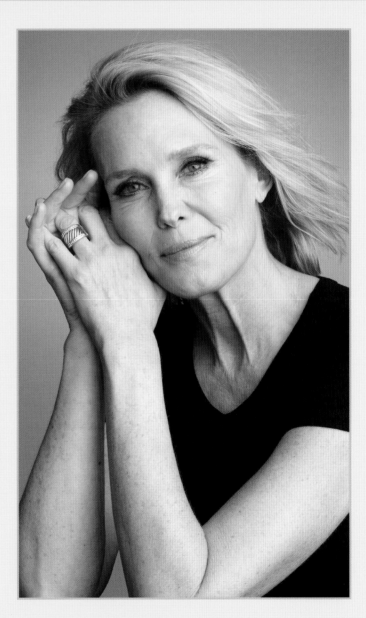

The Saggy Brow

If you're open to having work done, you have two options here: Botox or surgery. Botox works effectively and is the most popular choice. It eliminates the need for a browlift in many cases if you're willing to keep up a maintenance schedule every couple of months. Surgery is the solution if you don't want to be Botox dependent or your degree of sag can't be helped by Botox alone. Sometimes a descended brow pushes the eyes downwards in a domino effect, so you have droopy brows and saggy lids, too.

Dr. Daniel Baker says: "Browlifts are way overdone in terms of number of procedures and the elevation of the brow to an unnatural level that looks done. This procedure has dropped off 50 percent lately because Botox is taking care of the problem for many women in a more natural way."

Dr. Patricia Wexler says: "If you start using Botox in your brow area during your thirties, it's possible to prevent the need for a browlift later on. By preventing the muscle from moving, you're also preventing laxity from developing. However, the minute you do Botox between the brows (to treat perpendicular furrows called the elevens), it also pushes a crease up into the hairline. When a woman has a high forehead and significant laxity, I say it's time for an endoscopic brow lift.

You can also inject filler like Restylane in the deep plane parallel to the brow to give the brow a lift and arch lasting four to six months."

Dr. Fredric Brandt says: "I rarely recommend a browlift. Botox works extremely well to solve the issue of droopy brows and eyes if done correctly. Of course in some cases, especially if a woman is much older and the degree of sag is extreme, a browlift could provide a solution; but it leaves scars, looks obvious, and you do experience hair loss no matter what anyone says."

SANDY +LOIS *say:*

Botox affects brow shape. Wait a week after you have your Botox done before getting your brows shaped or tweezing yourself at home. The brows will be in a different position. Consider Botox as a solution if you have severe brows with a strong, sharp arch that give your face an angry expression. And definitely do Botox if you're plagued with perpendicular furrows between the eyes. It will paralyze the muscle for three months and your brows will be softer, more elongated, and make your pencil work easier to do.

Thanks, but no browlifts or Botox for now. What can makeup do?

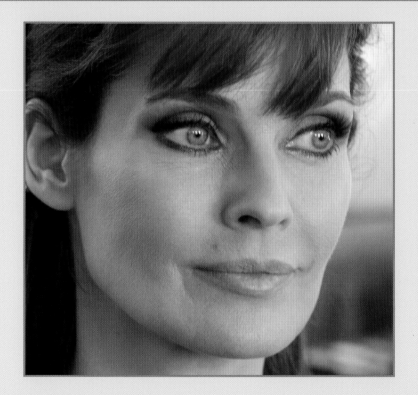

Be sure the outer brows do not droop or curve around your eyes, even if it means tweezing the tails completely away. You can then reposition the brow and stretch it outwards with pencil or wax and powder. This really creates a lifted look. Follow Sandy's brow technique in Chapter 2. Cutting full bangs can also work wonders as camouflage for forehead wrinkles as you use makeup to shape new brows.

Tired, Saggy Upper Eyes

We think corrective surgery is a great option if your eyes always look fatigued and applying eye makeup has come to feel like such a drag that you're ready to give up on it entirely. We've both been there. Doing your upper lids changes your expression from exhausted to rested and gives you a bigger, smoother canvas for eye makeup. Surgery trims excess skin, fat, and/or muscle and hides the scars in the fold of the lids.

Dr. Daniel Baker says: "Eyelids heal well because the skin is thin and rarely forms keloids (excess scar tissue that creates a ridge). Upper eyelid surgery lasts anywhere from fifteen to twenty years and is one of the most effective de-aging procedures you can do. Women often combine an eyelift with a facelift. "

Upper eyelid surgery establishes a hollow and allows you to define the crease. Your eyes will look huge and you'll want to experiment with makeup. Although you can return to work in about ten days, complete healing of wounds takes longer and you will have extensive bruising. Leave yourself a two-week window for complete recovery if you want to keep this procedure totally private.

Thanks, but no eyelid surgery
for now. What can makeup do?

Deep-set eyes with an overhanging upper lid can be amazing and exotic, so don't rush out to fix them, especially if your under-eye skin is relatively smooth. Avoid contouring the crease because this will make your eyes seem even more recessed. Line the upper eye according to Sandy's eye lesson in Chapter 1, but add more definition with your liner beneath the eyes. Try a smoky look by smudging this pencil or retracing it with shadow liner. If you love lining the lower inner rims, this can work well too if don't have a "wet" inner eye (and some women do, in which case don't do this!). Use soft neutral eye shadows on the lids—no dark shadows.

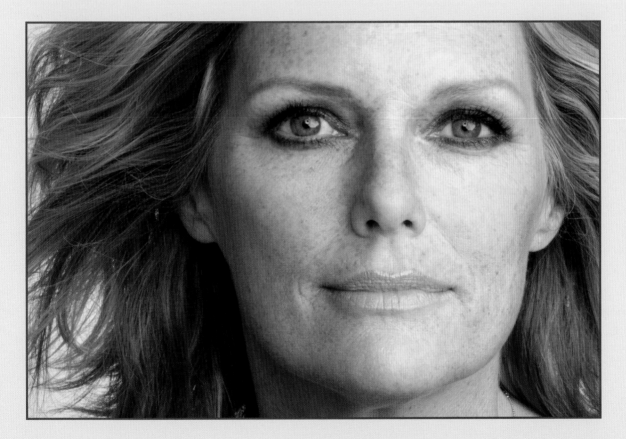

Under-eye Bags

Under-eye bags are often the result of genetics, but can be a structural issue too. In some cases the ligaments that support the fat pads around the eye weaken with age, causing the fat to slip and bulge forward. The skin in that area loses elasticity and the skin gets baggier as the pouch of fat balloons. Preparation H has been a cult solution whispered about for years, but frankly who wants to put a hemorrhoid ointment under their eyes? Corrective surgery can permanently remove under-eye bags, making your daily makeup far easier to do.

Dr. Patricia Wexler says: "Combining filler with another technique, such as a fractional Co2 Laser Combo, tightens the skin over the bag for additional results. Other techniques include Thermage, which delivers radio frequency waves to the deep tissue to stimulate new collagen production, and Ulthera, which uses fractional ultrasound to the same end result. Most important, do not remove the fat pad without lifting the mid face or ligament laterally; or injecting filler into the deeper plane. A hollow is not a substitute for a bag!"

Dr. Fredric Brandt says: "Under-eye bags can be eliminated permanently with surgery but fillers provide another option. Filling around the bags with Restylane or Perlane brings the recessed skin up to the same level as the bags. It's not permanent but it is an alternative solution for women who don't want surgery and want to look good for a specific reason, like job interviews, a high school reunion, or a wedding."

 SANDY +LOIS say: There are certain things makeup can correct in photos but not in real life. Under-eye bags are one of them. Big pouches cannot be taken away by any topical cream, no matter what the claims. Some women use a darker foundation or dark concealer on the swollen part of bags, but we think this makes the problem more obvious.

You are dealing with two issues here—skin color and skin texture. Get bags removed surgically if they are a problem, or at least get a consultation. Sometimes puffy under-eye bags cast a deep shadow near the tear trough, so you appear to have dark circles in addition to bags when in fact you don't. Once the bags are removed, the darkness vanishes too.

Thanks, but no eyelid surgery for now. What can makeup do?

Keep your upper eyelid makeup clean to compensate for loose skin and pouches below the eye and be sure to use an eye primer. You are not a candidate for the smudgy or smoky look. Your under-eye area should appear as bare and fresh as possible. Go easy on concealer— too much looks cakey and old.

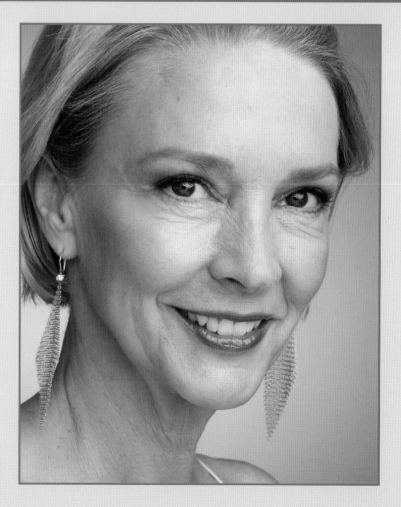

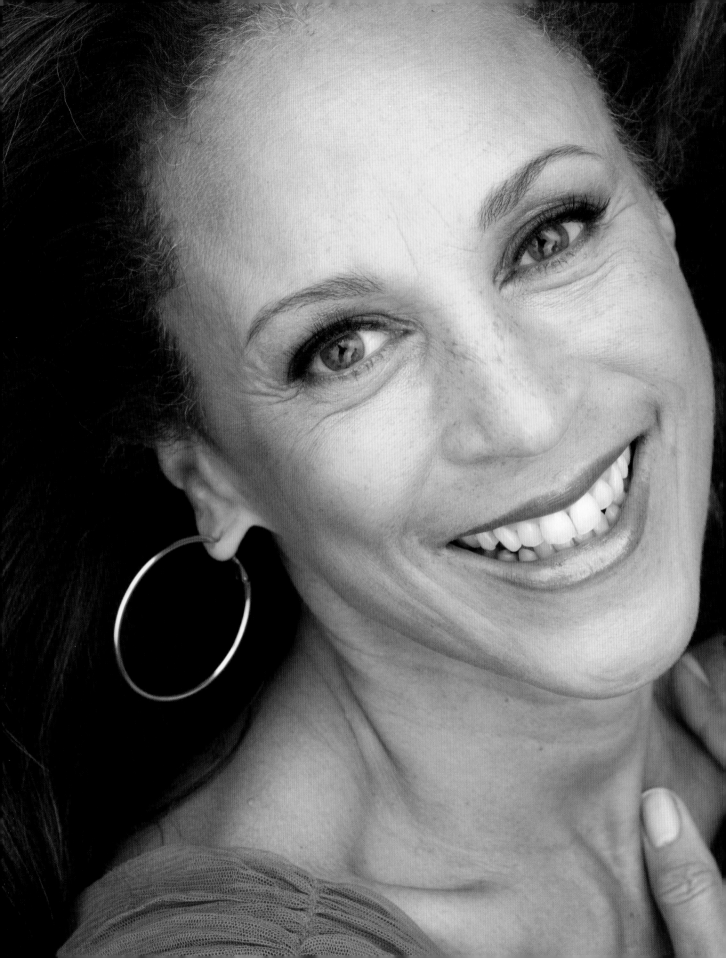

Saggy Cheeks +
Deep Nasolabial Folds

The nasolabial folds are the grooves that run from your nose to the corners of your mouth. Once they deepen and your cheeks drop, the folds make your lower face look heavy and saggy. Keep in mind that your face does not age with symmetrical precision either. One cheek will seem droopier, one nasolabial fold deeper, and the face can begin to look lopsided. By filling up the cheeks you can eliminate the sag and smooth out the nasolabial creases. Suddenly all anyone wants are high, round baby cheeks. Here are two different approaches by two top dermatologists.

Dr. Patricia Wexler says: "Cheeks are a question of aesthetics. A woman is never her most beautiful when her face is full in the middle (i.e. nasolabial fold). Filling the fold gives a bloated round face. Women want the widest point to be at the height of the cheekbones just under the eyes. What makes my aesthetic different is I do not believe in chiseling the lower part of the face, but a subtle transition from apple cheeks to jaw line. This gives the face a sexy youthfulness that sharp contouring does not."

Dr. Fredric Brandt says: "Restoring lost volume in the face is the real key to making your face look more youthful. Lots of women don't know this is what will make them look young. It's not about chasing every line. Fixing the one flaw you see in your magnifying mirror is not the answer. Saggy midface skin and a deep nasolabial fold is a symptom not a condition. It's a result of losing volume in the cheek area. If you fill only the fold you get heaviness in the lower face. If I use Perlane to build up the cheek, the fold gets lifted and smoothed out and the volume goes to the upper face, where it's most attractive. Most women examine their face from the front view only when considering fillers. If you inject the nasolabial folds only you will see a wave from the profile. You need to look at your face from all angles when making decisions about corrective filling or any work, including Botox."

SANDY +LOIS *say:*

Those deep nasolabial folds from nose to mouth are where your foundation tends to collect and crease. They can also add a sad or angry expression to your face. We've seen how effective a facelift or filling the cheeks can be in eliminating this problem. We think aiming for moderate fullness—not an extreme rounded face or big sculpted cheek—is the way to go. And a note of caution: some doctors inject silicone. We have seen bumps under the skin arise ten years later.

Thanks, but no fillers for now. What can makeup do?

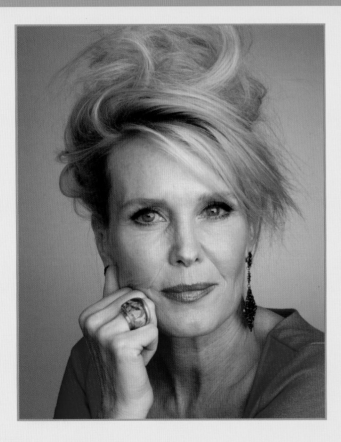

First of all, go lighter and sheerer with your foundation in these deep creases. Go over the area with a damp sponge after you finish your face to pick up any residue and repeat this trick to refresh your makeup during the day. As always, whenever lower face issues are the problem we say redirect the focus to your upper face with a stronger eye makeup and be sure to relocate your blush to the top of the cheekbone. Consider getting your teeth whitened—the prominence of this area deserves the de-aging effect a brighter smile delivers.

Thin, Flat Lips

Big, cushy pillow lips are everywhere. If good genes gave you a full, well-shaped mouth, we'll bet you're a lipstick lifer who loves to wear gorgeous colors (and still can). The fakes are obvious and sadly there's a rash of fifty-something women who have inflated their lips to a ridiculous degree. Lip filling is psychologically addictive, especially for women who never had full lips to begin with. Like bust enhancement, too many women are taking lips to an extreme. If done with a very subtle hand, filler can help restore volume and definition. The key words here are Very Subtle.

Dr. Fredric Brandt says: "Filled lips should blend with your face. They shouldn't be the first thing you see. Everything should be in proportion. Some women have their lips filled and then panic when the initial plumping and swelling goes down—which it will. They immediately assume they need to do more. Go slowly and find a responsible doctor who will keep the look natural and believable."

Dr. Patricia Wexler says: "Fat injections give the lips lift and volume that is graceful, not bumpy. But the real question women should be asking is: What is it that will give my face the most youthful rejuvenation? Frankly, I don't think its lips. I think its finding the right proportion of cheeks to jaw line and having clean, healthy-looking skin. But if you want lip augmentation, achieve definition and lift—the goal here is not volume."

 SANDY +LOIS *say:* Big, overdone lips are a dead giveaway. Unfortunately, some women don't ask for the lips they used to have but instead insist on getting someone else's lips. Whether you opt for hyaluronic acid or fat fillers, the results should not be obvious to anyone looking at you as "enhanced lips."

Fillers can correct lip asymmetry and restore definition to faded borders. If you have thin lips, the goal is to subtly plump them up so they don't vanish into your skin tone. The benefits of a good filler can actually make wearing lipstick easier and more appealing again. Bruising of the lips at the injection sites is sometimes a temporary problem and coverage can be difficult. Apply three thin coats of a deep matte lipstick with a brush, blotting between coats. Or, try using a deeper color lip pencil to color in the lips.

Be sure you go to a dermatologist or cosmetic surgeon who has extensive experience with lip filling and ask to see before and after photos or patient recommendations. This is frankly a painful procedure, though only at the moment of injection. Afterwards your lips may feel a little tight and seem swollen beyond your expectations. Ask your doctor how to minimize the discomfort and relax. Any excess redness or fullness will disappear in a week.

Thanks, but no fillers for now. What can makeup do for my thin, flat lips?

Use a lip-toned pencil to equalize your lip contours, especially any irregularities in the top bow. Fill in the lips with the same pencil and top with a shimmery gloss. Sometimes thin lips can look fuller if you join the cupid's bow into a rounded shape instead of drawing on points. This will also look more natural.

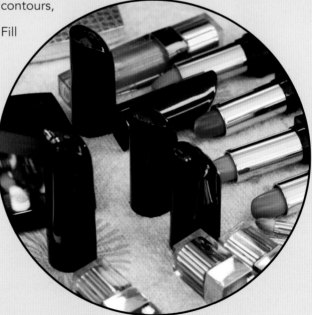

PRIVATE CONSULTATION ON YOUR
2 BIGGEST QUESTIONS

Q: As a skin doctor,
do you believe in makeup?

Dr. Patricia Wexler: "I've always worn makeup. I put lipstick on before going into my C-section! It's not about covering. Makeup is about enhancing the way you feel—not look, but feel. A little color brings life to the face. I feel invisible without it. As a redhead, with naturally pale brows and lashes, I need *something*—even if it's only brow pencil and mascara. Sandy is a friend, client, and my makeup artist too. When she makes me up for a big event, she uses my everyday makeup but just takes the intensity up a notch.

You need to stay current with makeup. The truth is, the older your skin gets, the less forgiving it is with makeup. The enemy of any fifty-year-old is oil-free foundation. Nothing makes wrinkles look worse than foundation that's heavy and matte. A tinted moisturizer is ideal for women dealing with extreme pigmentation and textural issues."

Dr. Fredric Brandt: "Once a woman starts doing fillers to restore volume, and using topical creams or lasers to get a smoother texture, she ends up with a fuller, firmer face that reflects light differently. You have a cleaner, tighter, fresher look and that changes your thinking about makeup. You cannot and should not look back and try to replicate the look you had five, ten, or twenty years ago."

Q: What are the biggest mistakes women make about their looks as they age?

Dr. Patricia Wexler: "I think the amount of Photoshop going on in magazines and advertising is giving women unrealistic expectations about their looks as they get older. Having some expression in your face is important. You can't—and shouldn't—freeze your expression lines away to nothing. The key to looking youthful is really about finding balance; keeping the right amount of expression, keeping the right proportion of filler and Botox; and having skin that is radiant, even in tone, and healthy.

No matter how much lifting and filling you do, if you have brown spots your skin looks old. Get rid of them! Sun damage can make skin look dirty and dull. Skin is a textural issue and you want it clear and radiant. Patients need to realize too that lasers change every six months and there are always new procedures with new names. They cannot and should not be trying and doing every new trend or filler that's on the market. Choose one filler and stick with it. There has to be a trust between doctor and patient when it comes to decisions about what to do and when to say, 'No thanks.'

Rejuvenation does not stop at the doctor's office. You are responsible too! Diet, hydration, and a daily regimen including moisture and SPF are essential! Avoid excessive alcohol, tobacco, and get more sleep. Be realistic. Don't get obsessive."

Dr. Fredric Brandt: "The biggest misconception women have about their looks comes from airbrushed magazine covers. Women see these Photoshopped images with no visible lines, pores, or textural changes and they measure themselves against that. Show more flaws! Stop judging yourself so harshly. Most women focus on little things they see in their magnifying mirror. They think getting rid of a line is going to make all the difference.

Looking youthful has a big psychological component. Women need to take responsibility for their health and looks by treating the exterior and the interior. You need inner health and confidence to complement the packaging."

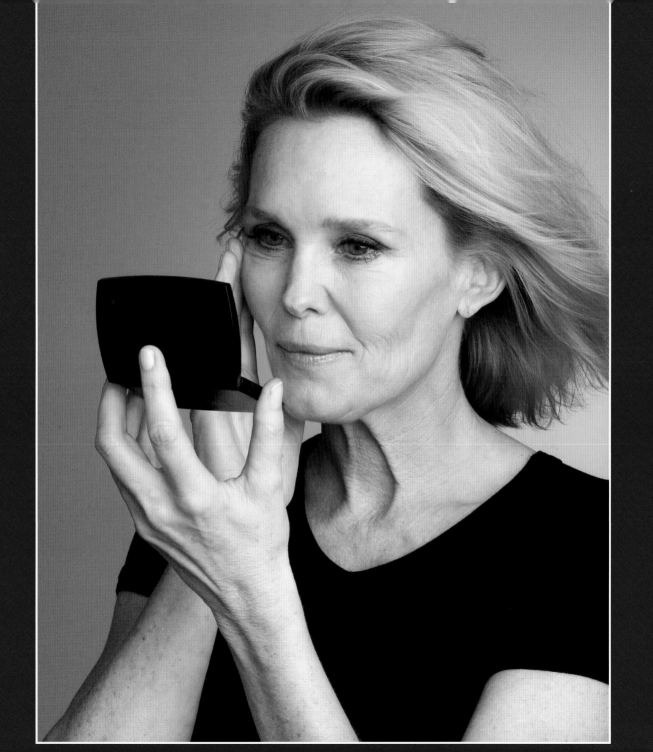

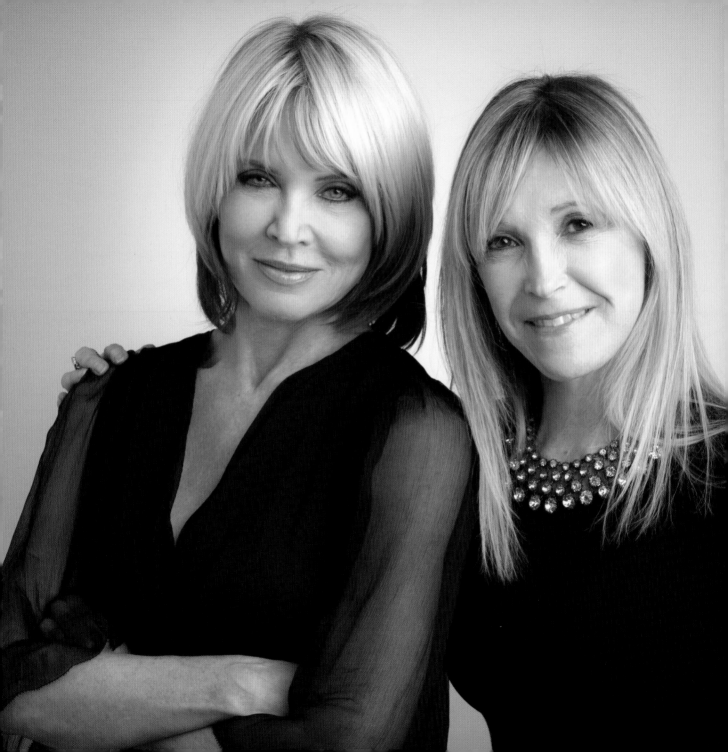

Sandy + Lois's current makeup and medical enhancement philosophy:

Sandy is a big believer in doing everything she can to improve her looks and maintain them. Here is her personal story: "I had my eyes done first at thirty-seven by Dr. Frederick Marks to remove under-eye bags when I realized the fortune I'd been spending on eye creams wasn't working. My bag problem happened gradually, but it interfered with wearing makeup. I wasted my entire thirty-sixth year prior to that first surgery trying to cure my puffy, baggy eyes by eliminating all salt and alcohol from my life. It got so I hated showing up on shoots with puffy under-eye bags. Dr. Marks convinced me to do both tops and bottoms. The results of that first procedure lasted until I turned sixty. By then I was looking crepey under my eyes and wanted to freshen up. This time, Dr. David Rosenberg did just the bottoms. He performed eyelid surgery and a chemical peel to my lower lid.

When I was forty-four, I went to see Dr. Patricia Wexler for the first time. I had been noticing my lipstick looked dry and cracked. The sides of my lips had shrunk, giving them a pursed look. Our mutual late friend, Bunny Kopelman, suggested I see Pat. The next week I was in her waiting room. She filled my lips with collagen, which looked natural and made me very happy. The filler also had a side effect I hadn't anticipated—it took away the dryness, my lipstick looked great, and it lasted longer.

The face ages asymmetrically. For instance, one brow can become lower than the other. Dr. Wexler corrected this issue for me, as well as the lines on my forehead, using Botox. I started doing Pat's makeup and she started doing my fillers and it became a client-client relationship and friendship that's lasted almost twenty years.

I had a facelift at forty-eight with Dr. Alan Matarasso, before the need for one became noticeable. At sixty-two I felt it was time to refresh and address the skin laxity in my neck so I had a second facelift, which was more intensive, with Dr. David Rosenberg. I did the second facelift before the need became noticeable."

Dr. Rosenberg says: "Sandy is a beautiful woman to start with. I did what I call my 'platysma muscle suspension facelift' on her. It's a modification of the deep plane facelift. This defined her jaw line and neck, and I repositioned the fat that had fallen back onto the bone to give the cheeks a higher, fuller look. It's what I call a very thorough facelift, and I didn't use any fillers to supplement the procedure."

Lois has a more laid-back approach to getting work done these days, but maybe that's because she had a serious bout of skin cancer in 2008: "Botox doesn't scare me; neither do scalpels. But Mohs surgery, the procedure for removal of skin cancer, sure does. Dr. Brandt found a basal cell carcinoma on the tip of my nose during a Botox procedure. I could easily be a Botox junkie because Fred Brandt does magic with that syringe. With a few well-placed jabs, my eyes look bigger and more open, my brows are lifted, and the cords in my neck vanish.

But once your nose is basically shaved off with Mohs and left to heal (I spent about a month and a half bandaged, feeling absolutely hideous), you begin to value health over perfection. Dr. Baker did the reconstructive surgery with a graft from my ear and it's a world-class nose now, but I'm cured of a knee-jerk attitude towards cosmetic surgery. Dr. Brandt zapped off the worst of my brown spots last year with liquid nitrogen. I still have crappy brows and my same original skinny lips though. But I've learned to do my very best with makeup cues from my chum, Sandy. For now I'll live with the problem areas. Stay tuned."

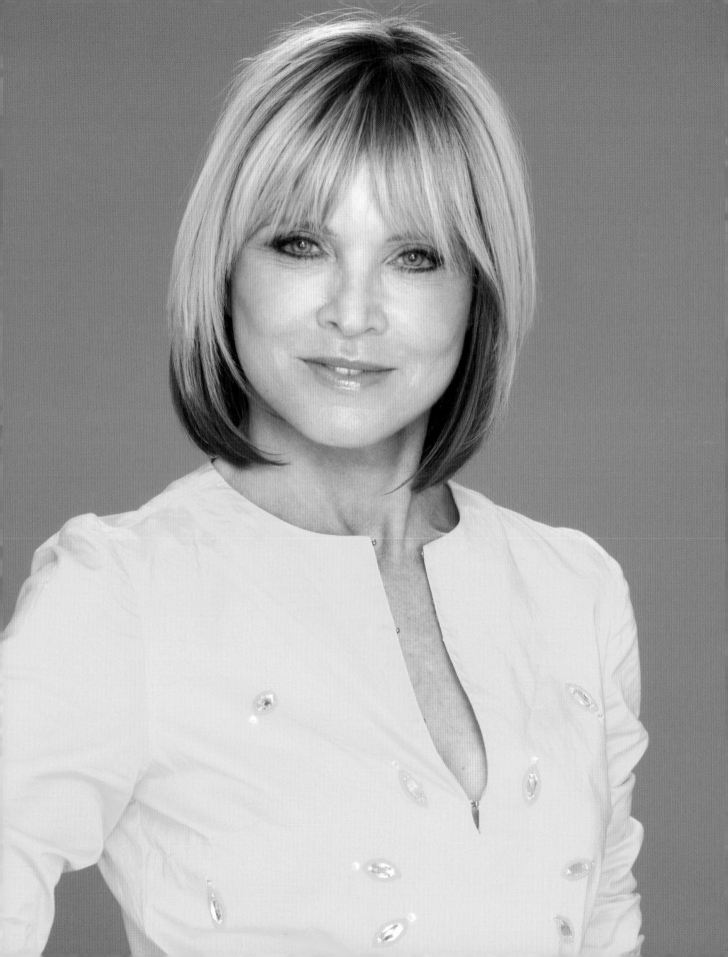

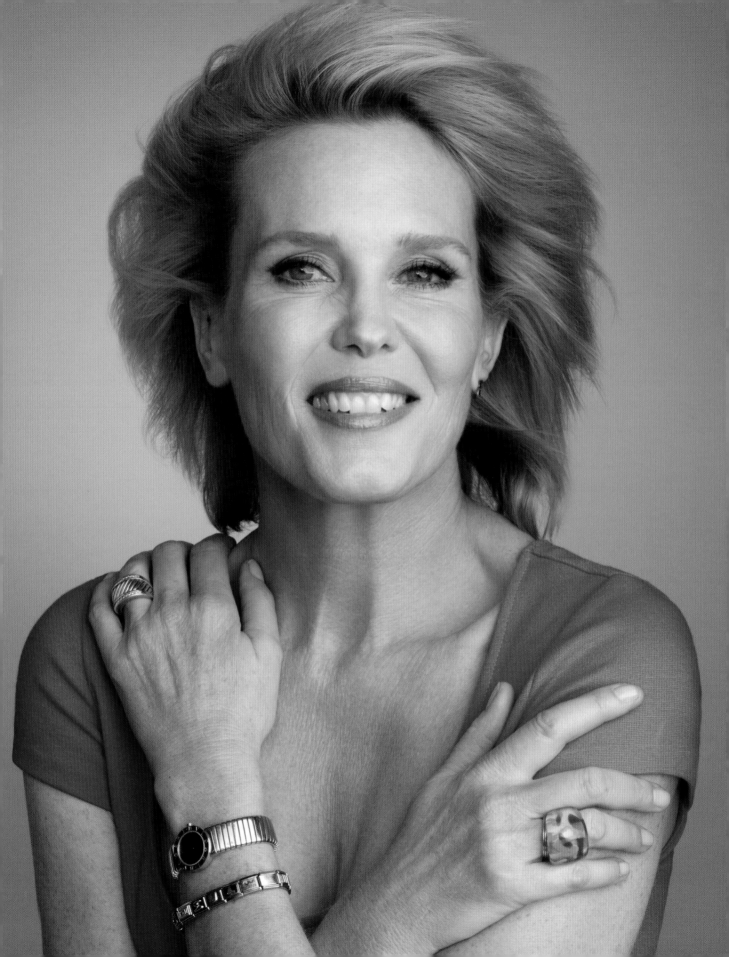

CHAPTER SIX

OBSESSIONS: DEALING WITH YOUR DEMONS!

Certain beauty topics are taboo— even among friends. Do you sneak into your local tanning salon and then pass off the head-to-toe bronze gleam as self-tanner? Do you Google "hair loss in women" and wear baseball caps all weekend? Do you wear extra long sleeves or gloves to hide your veiny, bony hands? Do you long to go bare legged in dresses but stick to cropped pants all summer to cover the spider veins and brown

Nancy Donahue

spots? We know all about tanning addictions, hormonal breakouts, spotty legs, crepey chests, hair loss, hot flashes that flip your face from glowing to greasy—and yes, the facial hairs framing your lip gloss. We all have our demons. Here are your dozen most heinous secrets and a way out for each. Think of us as your support group because we're here to share:

1. I'm a Tanorexic.

We are the first generation that took tanning seriously. We stocked up on sun reflectors, mixed baby oil and iodine as marinade, and wore the tiniest bikinis for maximum exposure. Now some of us can't let go. A tan was supposed to be sexy, make us look thinner, younger, and healthier. Fast forward a couple of decades and we now know a tan is not healthy. It's a sign of sun damage to your skin. A tan does not hide cellulite or make you look glamorous. That's pure beauty BS. Tans are dangerous. And don't think you're safe if you have naturally dark skin. Women of African American, Asian, Latino, Middle Eastern, Native American, East Indian, and Mediterranean descent get skin cancer too.

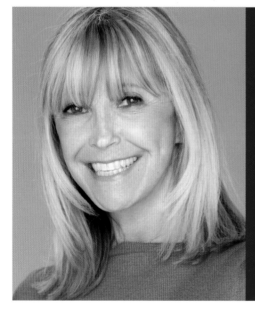

The allure of a tan is hard to break, but tanning is skin crack and if you're still doing it now, consider yourself a tanning junkie. Those summers are showing up thirty years later as wrinkles, brown spots, saggy skin, and skin cancer. And don't fool yourself; makeup won't make up for the damage.

So why are women who certainly know better sneaking into tanning salons for a hit of UV or skipping sunscreen during the summer (just this once)? We know a tan feels good. UV rays do trigger the release of the feel-good brain chemicals called endorphins. After a summer of tanning or routine sun-bed tanning, stopping cold turkey can cause withdrawal symptoms. Big deal. Get those endorphins through a workout or a fast walk instead. Don't talk yourself into thinking tanning is essential for Vitamin D, or that it prevents seasonal affective disorder (SAD) in winter. It doesn't to any extent that justifies prolonged sun exposure.

Lois says:

I have naturally fair skin and grew up near the beach on Long Island. I wore white shirts to school after vacations to show off my tan, which was actually the color of a barbecued chicken. I'd get blistering sunburns during the summer and have to deal with the peeling afterwards, but that didn't deter me from frying. I wanted skin that was a sunny, caramel color, like the models in *Vogue* and *Glamour* had.

Now, three years after a basal cell carcinoma and serious skin cancer reconstructive surgery on my nose, I'm totally anti-tan. I think tanning shows a lack of responsibility for your body and your health. If you still tan you're in denial. While the basal cell carcinoma I had is rarely fatal, it can be extremely disfiguring. Look up Mohs surgery online if you need to scare yourself into staying out of the sun!

If you're between the ages of forty-one and fifty-nine, you've already had more than 70 percent of your lifetime sun exposure. If you're between sixty and seventy-eight, the number zooms to near 100 percent. Approximately 68,720 melanomas—the deadliest form of skin cancer—are diagnosed each year. The survival rate for early detection is about 99 percent. Please get annual total face and body skin cancer checks, even if you opt out of any

According to the Skin Cancer Foundation, more than one million skin cancers are diagnosed each year and contrary to popular belief, 80 percent of your sun exposure is not acquired before the age of eighteen; it's only about 20 percent.

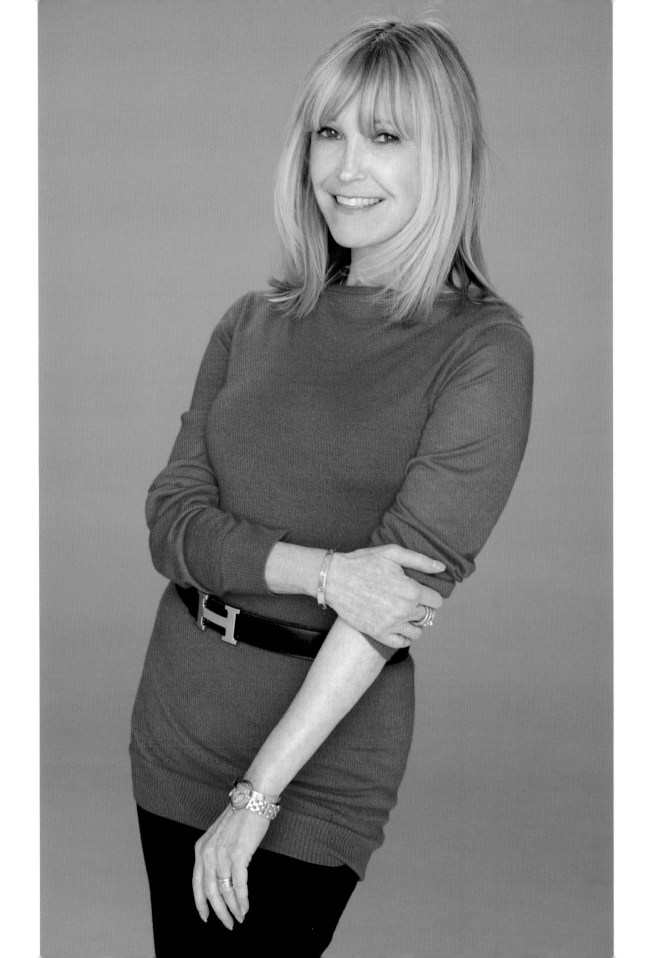

dermatological procedures. Still hooked? Ask your doctor if she has a UV camera to show you the age spots and pigmentation changes lurking beneath and not yet visible to the naked eye. Dermatologist Dr. Fredric Brandt helped me dodge a bullet when he diagnosed my skin cancer in 2008.

How can I wear full sunscreen and makeup and not compromise either one?

 If you have skin cancer issues, like I do, you always need an additional sunscreen of SPF 30 under makeup—even if the makeup itself has sunscreen. For adequate protection you need a full teaspoon of sunscreen for the face. I find the new light, non-greasy matte sunscreens compatible with makeup. Remember, if you plan to spend the day outdoors (whether you're on a cycling tour in Tuscany or just shopping at a flea market), you need to reapply sunscreen every two or three hours—even over makeup.

If you can't let go of your tan obsession, at least switch to self-tanners and bronzer. Just be aware that any self-tanner will also darken your brown spots. Don't attempt or expect to go from Meryl Streep pale to Vanessa Williams tawny. A fake tan that's too dark and unnatural is aging. Respect your own natural skin tone and aim for a slightly warmer version and get just a hint of a sunny glow. Gradual self-tanners that work slowly and progressively are the best choice because they give you more control over the color.

If you self-tan your face or wear bronzing powder, a progressive self-tanner applied neck to toes can help create a seamless, natural look. Otherwise you end up with a tanned face and pale hands, chest, and legs. You'll still get a feel-good lift and then can follow Sandy's makeup bronzing lesson in Chapter 4 to finish the look.

 Dr. Patricia Wexler has removed pre-cancer lesions from my chest area every few years. She also removed a deeper one next to the bridge of my nose, which I was told to keep an eye on.

2. I live in opaque tights or pants, long sleeves, and high neck tops . . . just to hide my brown spots.

We're not referring to a sprinkle of pinpoint freckles that were cute at ten. It's those large dots, or clusters of brown pigment that began sprouting after forty that make us cringe. We call them brown spots now but they used to be called age spots, or worse yet, liver spots due to their slug-like color. An opaque concealer in a peachy-apricot shade can successfully camouflage a couple on the face (see Sandy's camouflage method in Chapter 3).

Once the spots become larger or darker or increase in number you need a foundation with fuller coverage and dermatological help. Brown spots can discolor your chest, hands, and legs too and they become more visible in color and quantity each year. They can eat away at your confidence and wardrobe options. Laser removal is advisable for larger areas, liquid nitrogen for random spots.

We are fortunate to have two iconic models, Cheryl Tiegs and Patti Hansen, pictured in this section. During the height of their careers, both Cheryl and Patti were asked to sit in the sun and bake, tanning themselves for three days prior to swimsuit photo shoots. With proper care, these women managed to reverse the effects of sun damage and they look amazing.

Let's ask the doctors. What's the cutoff point?

Dr. Patricia Wexler says: "Most women are asking for rejuvenation of the face and neck as a unit because where do you define the anatomic boundary when it comes to aging skin? If you do the neck and face without doing the chest, what happens when you wear a low-cut dress or a deep V neck?"

Dr. Fredric Brandt says: "You can remove all your brown spots from your face to the top of your bra, or just get the major ones; it depends on how compulsive you are. If you're going to be spending a lot of time in the sun because say, you're a golfer, forget trying to remove all your brown spots. They'll be back. Freezing with liquid nitrogen still gives excellent results, especially when done in a series. Or, you can have a laser take care of them instead."

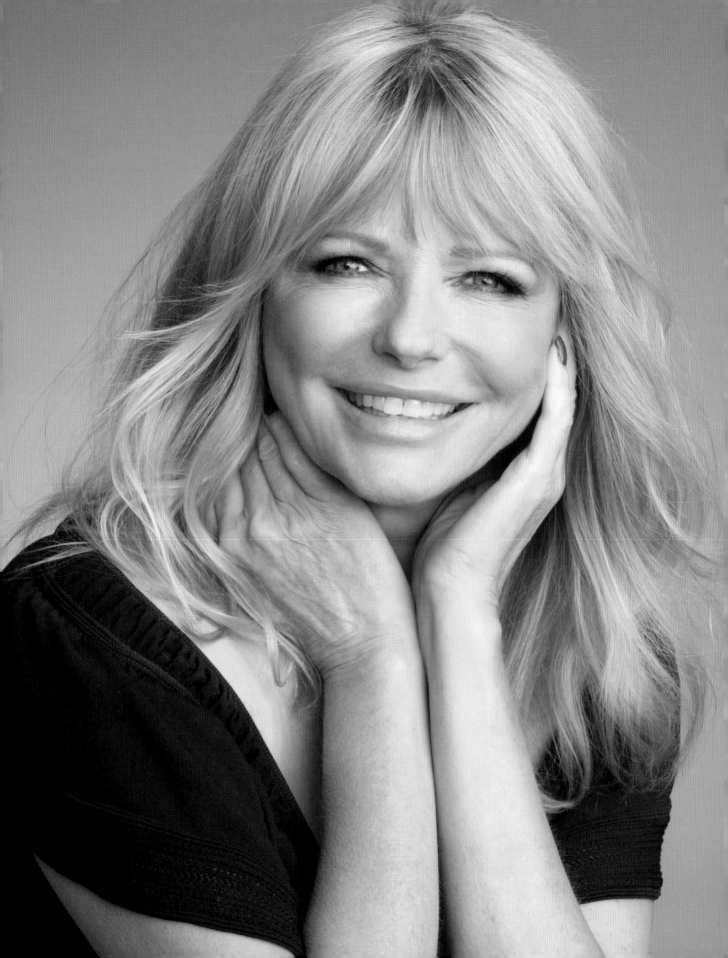

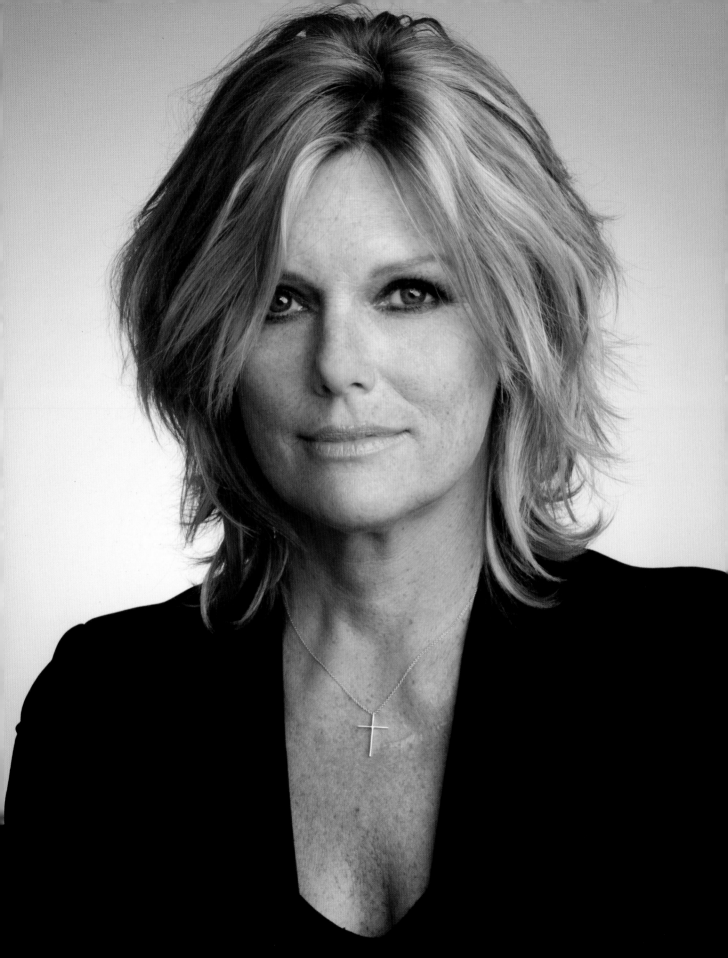

We think if you opt for dermatological treatment of brown spots, deciding how far to take the removal process depends on your fashion style and your lifestyle. Do you go to the office year-round in sleeveless knee-length sheaths that reveal your bare arms and legs? Do you live in Miami, Arizona, or Texas and spend most of your time out-doors? Would you wear more scoop-neck tops and draped necklines if you didn't have a spotty chest? (And while we're on the subject of cleavage, did you know spotty, crepey cleavage can be injected with Botox to smooth out that area too? Just FYI.)

Thanks, but no dermatological treatments for now.
What can makeup do to camouflage brown spots on my chest and legs?

To camouflage random major brown spots on your chest or neck, just tap on a water-resistant opaque concealer like CM-Beauty by Cover Mark Coverstik or Dermablend Quick Fix Concealer SPF 30. I do this whenever I'm wearing V-necks, scoop-neck dresses, or a camisole under a jacket. A foundation spray designed for legs, like Sally Hansen's, is ideal for quick coverage when you're wearing bare legs to the office. For serious coverage I like Dermablend Leg and Body Cover Foundation. This is opaque and waterproof and needs to be applied sparingly. Although my legs are pretty good I have spider veins, brown spots, and dozens of pinpoint red dots that make me reluctant to shed my nude fishnets in summer. The extra coverage makes summer weekends in the country, swimming, and wearing sundresses and flip-flops easy.

Sally Hansen Airbrush Legs does a great job with non-transferable color and should be enough for everyday wear. You can even use it on your chest. I used to apply sunscreen to my face but not my chest and as a result had sun damage in that area. I had all precancerous cells cut off and biopsied and my brown spots lasered off by Dr. Patricia Wexler.

3. Uh-oh. I forgot about my hands.

We hear this a lot. Sometimes there was nothing you could have done to avoid it. Bony hands with prominent veins and loose skin are inevitable signs of aging. Brown spots on the back of your hands are a sign of sun damage. Some women were super smart about applying sunscreen and moisturizer to their faces, but let their hands slip through the cracks. Spotty hands are even more annoying if you've spent time and money eliminating brown spots from your face and chest. To prevent further damage and restore softness, wear a sunscreen on your hands every day and reapply it often. Even if you're just gripping the steering wheel while driving, your hands are vulnerable to UVA rays. They come straight through glass.

Let's ask the doctors for their take on hands that give away your age.

Dr. Fredric Brandt and Dr. Patricia Wexler say: "There are two great dermatological solutions to rejuvenate aging hands. Get filler injected into the back of your hands to restore a youthful smoothness and hide veins, then get a laser treatment to remove the brown spots. Maintain with regular exfoliation, topical rejuvenation (like retinol), and SPF daily in your moisturizers."

Good to know, but no lasers for now.
What can I do myself if my hands look older than my face?

Your hands are victims of the same changes that show up on your face—moisture loss, uneven pigmentation, and a slowdown in cell renewal. Fillers do give your hands a supple, young look. They raise the skin just enough so veins and bones are not the focus of attention, and lasers can vaporize brown spots.

There are things you can easily do yourself to improve your hands though. Start applying sunscreen to the backs of your hands every day. You'll be preventing further sun damage. Stash hand cream in your bag, desk, car, bedside table, and by every sink.

Look for those that have de-aging ingredients like retinols, AHAs, skin-lightening botanicals, and antioxidant vitamins like A and E, in addition to moisturizers and humectants that keep hands soft.

Do regular microdermabrasion at home or in the doctor's office to get rid of dead skin cells and yes, you can use the same one you use on your face. Different microdermabrasions recommend different frequency of application. Cell turnover is essential to achieving brighter, younger skin. We suggest keeping your nails on the short side simply because it looks more youthful, especially if you have pronounced knuckles or dry, tough cuticles.

We're also big fans of Deborah Lippmann's sexy polishes, and the hottest seasonal colors from Essie and OPI. Red is always a good option if you prefer a classic or retro look. For big emergencies when your hands are on show (lunch with clients, a date, a job interview), we suggest you get a salon paraffin wax treatment and a pro manicure, and be sure to dab opaque waterproof concealer on major brown spots.

Go for a fabulous nail color. It's the one place you can stay super-trendy and edgy in color cosmetics. Sheer beiges and naturals are tasteful but aren't going to do you any good. Color on the nails diverts attention away from the backs of your hands and pulls it towards your fingers and rings.

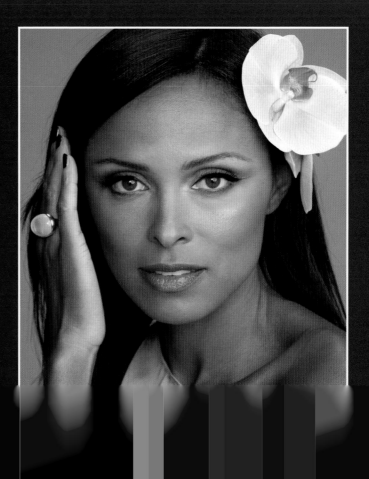

4. I have a mustache, less hair on my head, and my brows are half-gone! What's going on?

What does hair have to do with makeup? Everything. It frames your eyes and face to enhance them and works with your makeup to give you a youthful look. Let's not forget a full head of hair and full brows are also sexy—which is why time spent on them is time well spent.

When things flip flop and your locks start thinning, your hairline recedes, your brows vanish, and the only thing sprouting are dark hairs along your lip line, you need help. Menopause is usually the culprit. When the female hormone estrogen decreases, some women experience an increase in male hormones called androgens. The result can be a hairier upper lip and skimpier hair on your head. It's not always estrogen though. Each hair shaft normally gets skinnier with age. You may have the same number of hairs, but your overall texture can feel much thinner. Right about this time we notice our brows have thinned or started to disappear too.

Let's ask the doctors about hair and brow loss.

Dr. Fredric Brandt says: "Post menopausal hair loss and brow loss are two of the biggest concerns of older women today. If you're losing your brows, especially the outer halves, go get your thyroid tested immediately. I see a lot of women who are hypothyroid and have no idea there's a genuine medical reason and solution."

Dr. Patricia Wexler says: "The prescription drug Latisse is often helpful in restoring fullness to skimpy lashes, and it may help brows as well. Truly extreme brow loss can be helped by a brow transplant. Hair loss on your head in certain cases can be helped by a transplant, too. For women with hair loss mainly along the front hairline and top, but with thick hair in back, a hair transplant can be the solution. This is a surgical procedure where strips of scalp are removed and single hairs are grafted to fill in sparse areas in the front. Only a small percentage of women are candidates for this since it works for localized balding, not allover thinning. You need a surgeon who specializes in this procedure. (Contact the American Society of Plastic Surgeons and the American Society of Dermatologic Surgery for guidance in your area.)

OK, but suppose there are no medical issues and I don't want a transplant. What can I do?

Dark mustache hairs, even a handful, interfere with face and lip makeup. And yes, people do focus on it when you speak instead of that dazzling smile and gorgeous new lip gloss. Ask your doctor if you are a candidate for laser hair removal on the upper lip. There are still the options of bleaching, waxing, or electrolysis, too.

For women with allover thinning hair, we empathize. Every woman we know says she doesn't have the hair she had at twenty or thirty. For a cosmetic fix that really works, stick to a haircut that's somewhere between chin and collarbone length. Then use color and highlights to bulk up the hair shaft and add dimension. Color itself physically coats the hair shaft, so each strand actually increases in texture and gives your hair an overall thicker look. Highlights can diffuse the contrast between your visible scalp and hair. Gray roots always make your hair look thinner. Don't be lazy about color! Meanwhile, beef up those brows with Sandy's brow lesson in Chapter 2.

5. But my skin was fabulous up until menopause . . .

No question about it. When your estrogen goes, your skin gets thinner, drier, looser, and more lined on the surface. When the collagen and elastin support system in your skin collapses, your face sags like a mattress that's lost its stuffing and springs. It doesn't happen overnight though it may feel that way (stress and lack of sleep exacerbate lines and that saggy look). You now have a very different skin than you did decades ago and it's going to react differently to makeup. You need a new support system of skincare to pull ahead.

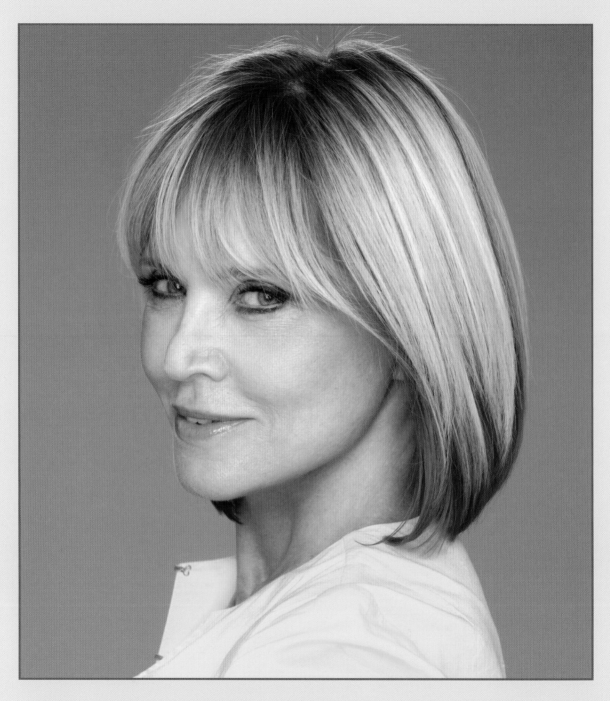

Sandy says: The day I went off Hormone Replacement Therapy (HRT) at the insistence of my doctor, the skin on my body totally collapsed. I am accepting it. The medical risks are not worth the skin benefits.

Wouldn't it be easier to just go back on HRT?
It did do great things for my skin. Let's ask the doctors:

Dr. Fredric Brandt says: "Look, HRT does do great things for the skin when women are menopausal. It brings back the thick, firm, plump texture. I know this is a huge issue now, but it all comes down to quality of life."

Dr. Patricia Wexler says: "You don't have to be on HRT to have great skin. We can supplement from the outside what you are missing from the inside. Improved skin is not a sole reason to be on HRT! Everyone benefits from a balanced diet, lots of water, and a multi-vitamin. Oral antioxidants are good to prevent internal malignancy like colon cancer."

While not all women experience wrinkles, loss of density, and dryness in equal amounts, every woman we've met complains about dehydrated skin when it comes to makeup application after menopause. So we have to ask, is your skincare routine doing its job for the face you have now?

Menopause can make your skin look fragile and translucent, and possibly dry, rough, uneven, matte, and wrinkled. The upper epidermal layer, the protective barrier of the skin, has thinned, and so have the middle dermal layer and the fat beneath. Your face can look flabby and untoned, making any wrinkles you have more noticeable. You can restore thickness with fillers at the dermatologist, but you need to do your homework, like changing your foundation and working on your application techniques.

You really do need to change or adjust your product usage to get better makeup results post-menopause. Hydrating the skin, rebuilding collagen for a firmer look, smoothing out lines, and evening out skin discolorations are achievable goals no matter what state your skin is currently in. Look for proven de-aging hero ingredients like retinols and acids (AHAs, BHAs, PCAs) that speed up skin cell turnover and smooth lines. They also make fresher cells appear on the surface.

At-home enzyme peels or acid cleansers also help buff away dead cells so that the surface of your skin looks cleaner and healthier. Vitamin C, peptides, and MMP inhibitors stimulate collagen production so skin can regain a firmer look. Hyperpigmentation fighters, like Vitamin C, azelaic acid, kojic acid, licorice root extract, and willow bark extract, can help mute or erase brown spots. Concentrated hydrating serums with a cocktail of the most current hi-tech de-agers put back that moist, dewy feel. And products that restore the skin's protective barrier, such as niacyl and EFAs, help prevent dehydration.

Oh, and one of the best things you can do to help yourself now is shut off your Blackberry and computer after 9pm! Menopausal women say they hardly sleep. That's a huge reason their skin looks dull, puffy, and fatigued, and making it up in the morning gets harder.

6. Will my new makeup make me breakout? How come I have pores like a teenager now?

When your hormones go awry during peri-menopause you feel sixteen again—and certainly not for any good reason. Giant pores and breakouts are not what we had in mind for our sophisticated years. Suddenly the pores on your nose and chin look like craters due to clogs of excess oil and sluggish dead cells. Exposed to air, this crud oxidizes and can turn into blackheads that make your skin look dirty and grimy even with the most perfect makeup.

Indoctrinated in our twenties to the words *oil-free*, *noncomedogenic*, and *dermatologist-tested*, we still worry that new makeup will trigger pimples—even at fifty! Well to be honest, it is possible an allergic reaction to certain ingredients can result in breakouts. It's also possible that hormonal changes, like the downshifting to low on estrogen and high on androgens, can cause acne. Any ingested drug that raises hormone levels, like lithium, birth control pills, or steroids, can trigger breakouts too.

Have a topical salicylic acid or benzoyl peroxide spot fix on hand, but select one designed for grownups with dry skin and zits. Topical prescription drugs derived from Vitamin A drugs, like

Retin-A and Renova, may turn out to be your ultimate solution. They treat wrinkles and breakouts, improve the shedding cycle of skin cells, prevent backed-up pores, and reduce inflammation.

What do the dermatologists have to say about this?

Dr. Patricia Wexler says: "I like Oracea, which is an oral antibiotic that has an anti-inflammatory effect, or the Isolaz laser for breakout-prone skin 40+. Isolaz unclogs pores and treats wrinkles at the same time. It's done in a series of treatments using suction methods to clean out your pores while pulsed light zaps oil and bacteria. Since there's no oil or cell buildup, Isolaz can also discourage blemishes. Aldactone is another adult acne fighter that has the added benefit of also treating hair loss. In-office microdermabrasion or light glycolic peels can improve pore texture, enhancing the work you do at home during your exfoliating routine.

Why these issues at this age? Years of sun damage to elastic tissue cause pores to enlarge. Self-tanners are infamous for causing breakouts and adding an SPF to face makeup can also cause blemishes. Rosacea is adult acne which can flare up too at this time in life. Check in with your dermatologist for your personal solution."

Dr. Fredric Brandt says: "Are you smoking or even 'sneaking' cigarettes? If you do, one thing—Stop Smoking! Aside from the obvious health issues, smokers have the worst pores. After menopause, sebaceous glands slow down and your skin gets drier even as your pore size increases. Smokers add self-destructive behavior to a natural process. Smoker or not though, if enlarged pores are getting in the way of their makeup, I tell patients to apply a mattifying primer first in those areas."

Clean up those pores—but *no squeezing*! There are two solutions to get rid of clogged pores yourself. Try at-home exfoliating products that list glycolic, salicylic, or lactic acid as a key ingredient. Or, try an enzyme mask that contains pineapple, bromelain, or pumpkin. Either way your goal is to loosen or dissolve dead cells to reveal the fresher skin beneath.

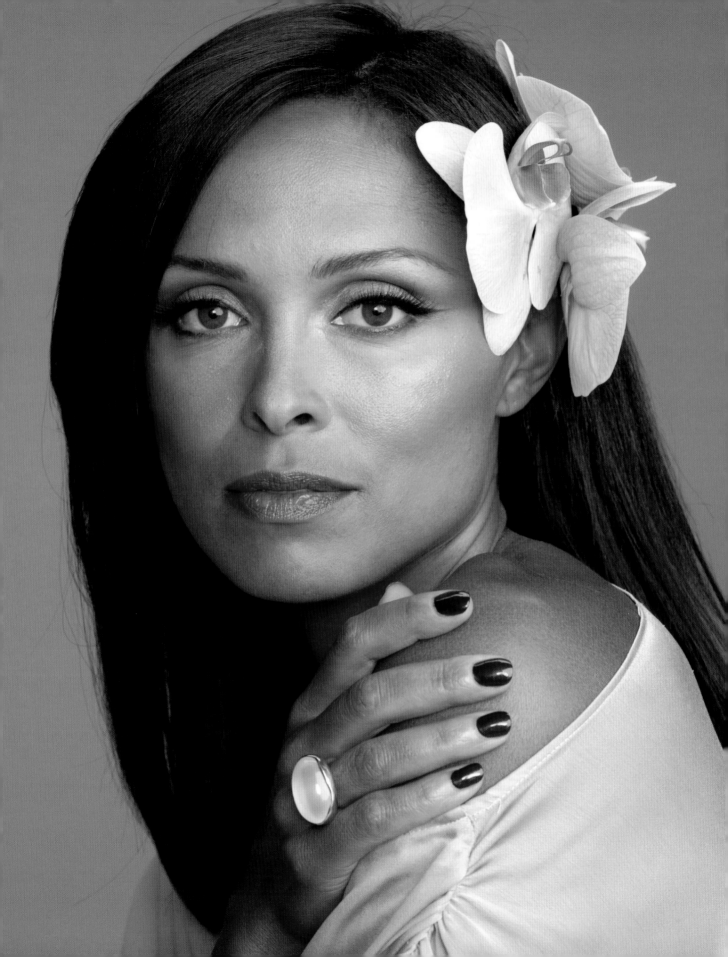

It's time to stop using pore strips made for teens with oily skin. They're not good for very dry or thin skin or retinoid, AHA, or BHA users. Instead, try a mattifying lotion under your makeup like Clé de Peau Beauté Oil Balancing Essence or a La Mer Oil Absorbing Lotion. And stop blotting. It's not oily skin anymore; it's glow.

And it should go without saying you take off all your makeup at night with a makeup remover to get every last bit of makeup out of your pores!

7. I never feel polished. What am I missing?

"I want to look polished" is one of the biggest requests Sandy hears from private clients. It's all about staying on top of the details. Polish really means paying attention to being well groomed and up to date. Perfecting your makeup application is part of the big picture, but it's only a start. First of all, forget about looking bohemian and natural. These are the words magazines use for a "straight-from-the-beach-or-bed" look that works when you're in your twenties or thirties. The so-called windblown, healthy good-looks pictures of stars or models in certain catalogs and ads are actually meticulously crafted.

What's charming and bohemian on a twenty-five-year-old is just messy, splotchy, and dirty when you're fifty. Looking polished is one of the perks and part of the power of being your age. Looking polished is the best revenge.

There's a to-do list of certain things that fine tune your appearance and lift it from careless to cared-for. Money can't buy polish, but women with money usually have it. Polish is about dedication to wiping out every flaw from hangnails to roots, crusty elbows to droopy ear piercings. Anyone can have polish; it just becomes routine. Here are ten things to get you started:

1 **Schedule in manicures or file, shape, and buff your nails to a rosy gleam.** Chips, raggedy over-grown cuticles, hangnails, or nails of mismatched, uneven lengths look sloppy. Skip the fakes like wraps, acrylics, and tips and aim for a modern, short, neat look.

2 **Keep your feet and toes sandal ready and "on call" all year long.** Corns, calluses, and blisters have just got to go. Make neat, smooth, healthy-looking feet and heels a must, not a maybe.

3 **Banish frizz. You can't have "wrinkled" hair *and* lines on your face.** Smooth, glossy, shiny hair makes your face look fresher. Keep it sleek with a salon keratin treatment, blow-outs prepped with straightening serums, and a backup kit of chic hair-toned ponytail elastics.

4 **De-crust your elbows, heels, and knees.** These three spots thicken with age and the pileup of dead skin cells can wreck the effect of elbow-length cardigans, knee-length dresses, and slingbacks. Use a body polish or scrub and major moisturizer daily—head to toe.

5 **Fix your torn or stretched ear piercings.** Earlobes lengthen, thin, and droop with age and if you're a fan of heavy or dangly earrings, those extended holes need repair by your dermatologist or cosmetic surgeon—and a redo a few months later.

6 **Get trims or at least dust the ends of your hair once a month.** Stay ahead of splits and stringy bits that separate like an old broom. Use hair masks to intensify hydration and shine at least once a week.

7 **If you are not gray, don't obsess about your roots.** Slightly darker roots can add a youthful look while perfect solid color, scalp to tips, can be aging.

8 **Smell heavenly.** Whichever scent you wear, be it Frederic Malle Carnal Flower or Guerlain Vetiver, it should smell classy, divine, and make people want to be near you. Carry a purse-size spray in your bag.

9 Never wear anything with stains, including bags and coats. Never wear hems with loose threads; sleeveless dresses with deodorant shadows; pilled sweaters; shoes or boots with worn heels; and clothes that no longer fit your current body, age, or lifestyle. That's what consignment shops are for. Whether your style is tailored, contemporary, artsy, or edgy, you still need to look crisp, clean, and put-together at all times.

10 Plan, don't panic—get a safe kit together. Have at your fingertips: your makeup essentials in a Ziploc baggie; statement jewelry, like earrings or a necklace to throw extra glow on your face; a mini dry shampoo mist to freshen yesterday's blow-out (or the day before); a top you feel gorgeous in to throw over jeans or a skirt; a cardigan in your best color; and amazing shoes you can actually walk in, like chic jeweled ballet flats.

8. Hot flashes make me a Sweat-er Girl.

When that sensation of steamy warmth creeps up your chest, neck, and face you're usually not in a sauna but at a meeting. For most women the feeling lasts only a few minutes, but in that time your face and scalp fill with perspiration, you flush, and you can feel your makeup begin to break down. That sudden sweaty feeling comes on when you least expect it. Water from the air plus your own sweat can leave your face feeling like glue.

Be prepared. If you're going through perimenopause and hot flashes frequently interrupt your workday or evenings out while wearing makeup, switch to transfer-resistant, all-day-wear foundations. These products require super-speed blending because they set quickly. Work from the back of the hand. Don't apply dots of foundation directly to your face. They dry too quickly and become difficult to blend. Most of them are oil-free or have a matte or semi-matte finish, and they deal effectively with extra moisture, especially during humid weather. All of these factors work in your favor. Some women tell us they also have great success with mineral powder makeup in the loose or powder compact versions for perspiration problems. We also recommend switching to matte, no-residue sunscreen, gels, or light, concentrated serums instead of heavy treatment creams. Carry blotting papers—and always use them before makeup application. Or, just take a quick bathroom break and run cold water over your hands and wrists.

9. Stained, dingy teeth limit my lipstick choices . . . and I smile with lips closed.

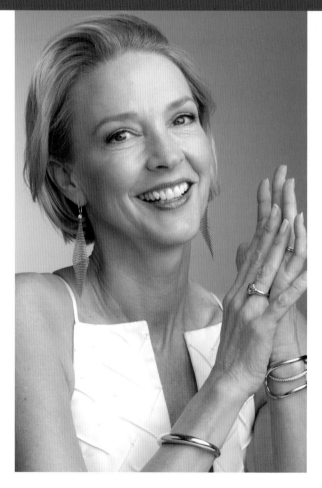

Tooth discoloration ultimately gets us all. Make that sooner rather than later if you smoke or drink red wine, coffee, or tea. No matter how fabulous your makeup, no matter how perfectly shaped your lips, if your teeth are yellow, forget it. Whiter teeth (even uneven ones) do look younger and are part of that groomed, polished look we all aspire to no matter what our stand on surgery or makeup. White teeth make thin, flat lips look fresher and healthier, and they amp up your lipstick choices, too. How many more reasons do you need?

Smile brightening is such an easy fix. You can opt for a dental procedure, at-home strips, or make an appointment with your dentist for an in-office bleaching, which can brighten your smile in one hour flat. Whitening trays custom-molded by your dentist or over-the-counter kits can help you maintain the results of bleaching. Get your old dark fillings replaced with tooth-color resin. It will make your fillings unnoticeable and can take years off your mouth, in addition to the whitening treatments or at-home strips.

Porcelain veneers or bonding, two other smile makeover options, can turn poorly spaced, discolored, chipped, or worn-down teeth into a movie star smile. Most celebs and models have these procedures done. Even doing the front four or six teeth makes a huge difference if your teeth are short or jagged. Veneers won't respond to bleaching, so bleach the teeth you are not doing them on before getting the veneers done and aim for a shade that blends. If you're like many women who are getting orthodontic braces in their forties or fifties to realign and straighten teeth that have shifted, opt for clear, virtually invisible braces like Invisalign.

And guess what? Improving the color, shape, and alignment of your teeth makes lips look fuller, your lower face more youthful, and of course opens up your choice of lipstick colors once again, too. If you haven't gotten around to whitening, lean towards lipstick shades that don't undermine or exacerbate the color of your teeth. Pass on vibrant reds. If your teeth are in the blue-gray range, cool pinks, berries, and roses on your lips can help counteract dinginess. If your teeth tend towards yellow, wear warmer lip colors in sunny nude, golden apricot, pink, or golden rose shades. Save the killer reds for the day you do get your teeth whitened.

10. Is it my hair color or my makeup that's off track?

We can show you how to use makeup to look your best, but what if your hair color isn't doing its job? The wrong hair color can drain color from your face, make you look sallow, or exaggerate lines and shadows. Color pro Brad Johns of the Brad Johns Studio at the Elizabeth Arden Red Door Salon in NYC says, "I always look at a client's makeup when we're discussing hair color. If she has started piling on the blush, or she's stepped up the self-tanning, or she's wearing a lot more makeup than usual, it's a tipoff that her color isn't working. I always look at a woman's eyes and skin and think

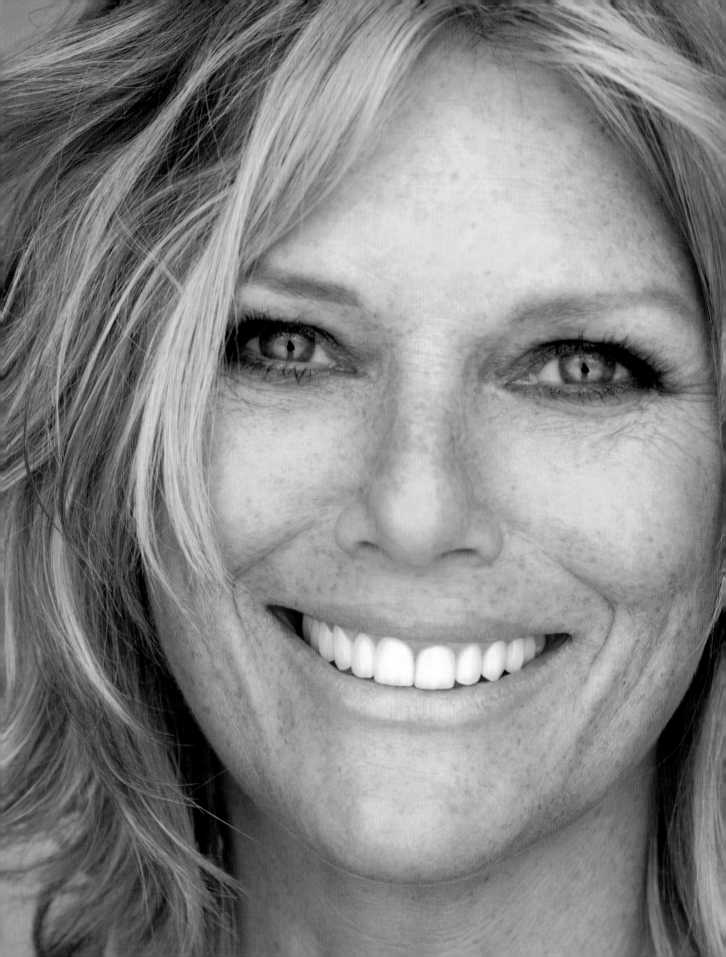

how can I make her shine more? I know it's time for a change when a client says she wants to go brighter because she feels drab."

As you age, your skin loses pigment and/or gains excess pigmentation in the form of brown spots, circles, and discolorations. This affects both your makeup and your hair color. If you change one, you need to address the other. They're partners in making the most of your looks. Brad says "Celebrities 40+ always go lighter or brighter, more dimensional and multi-colored, even if they stay brunette. It works better for them on camera, and that works for real life too. I like beachy hair color like Cindy Crawford's multi-tonal browns, or Ellen DeGeneres's short tousled crop. I think women who get on the improvement path change their hair color and makeup first and then go on to possible dermatological or cosmetic surgery procedures. They provide a big boost and you can modify hair color quickly and easily. But when someone gives you bad Botox or big, puffy, filled lips, you're stuck for awhile."

Any big change in your skin or makeup will affect your hair color. If you stop or start using self-tanner or bronzing powder, if you develop more brown spots, or if your skin starts looking blotchy or sallow, you need to rethink your hair color. You may need to go brighter, softer, lighter, or add highlights for a more multi-dimensional look. Discuss your changing skin tone issues with your colorist because that's where she can help. In general, brunettes need to lighten up as they age because the dark color can emphasize under eye shadows. Caution to blondes: don't go too blonde, too pale, or too solid in color. You need depth and a multi-tone color to look youthful.

Sandy says: If I am doing makeup on someone and their hair color is radically wrong, the makeup never looks as good as I want it to. I've been a victim of bad hair color myself. I had dark lipstick red hair and wanted to go blond but it turned orange. It was impossible for me to do my own makeup.

Kim Alexis

"I don't feel fifty—my mind is young and I feel healthy. I don't even wear glasses. Honestly, I don't think about my looks. About a year ago I cut my long, thick blonde trademark hair. I wanted something different—I was sick of always pulling it back in a ponytail and I wanted something short and layered but sexy. I'm pretty good at doing my own makeup by now. I don't like lip gloss at all; it's goopy. For my real life I wear long-wear lipsticks, like Revlon ColorStay; navy or black liner on the top lids; some Benefit concealer; and shadows in brown or gray for winter and shimmery gold for summer. I wish celebrities would go back to doing what they do best—acting—and I want to take back my covers and makeup and hair ads! Why aren't older models working to sell product? We really know how to do that better than anyone."

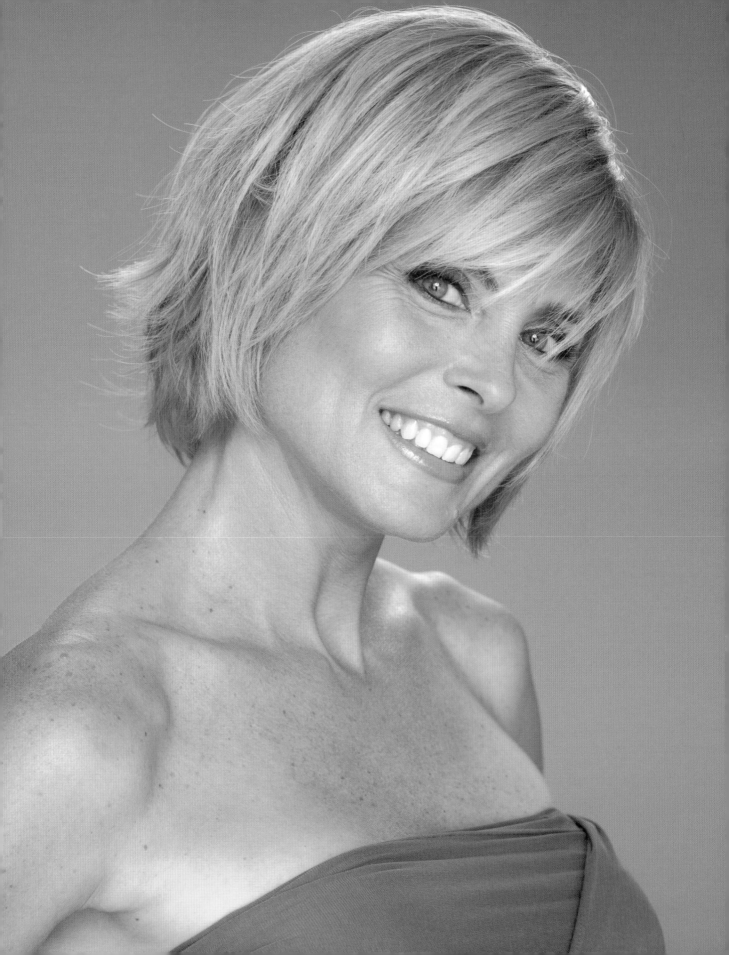

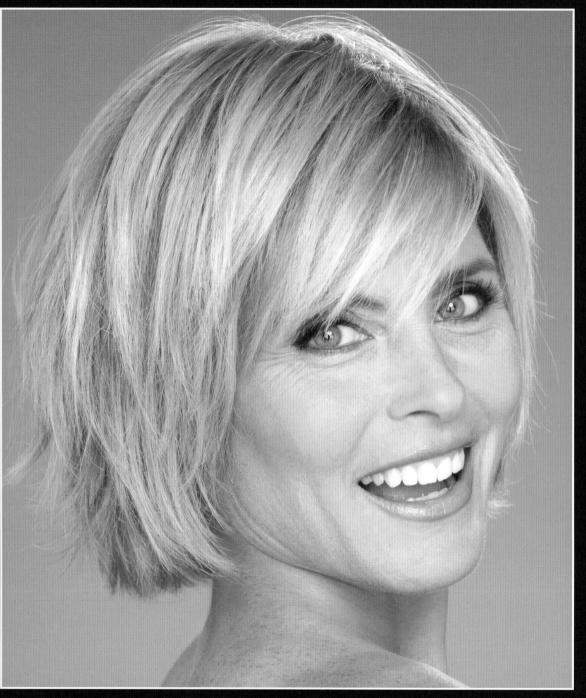

It's never one thing. The total package of hair color, cut, manicure, pedicure, skin care, and makeup work together.

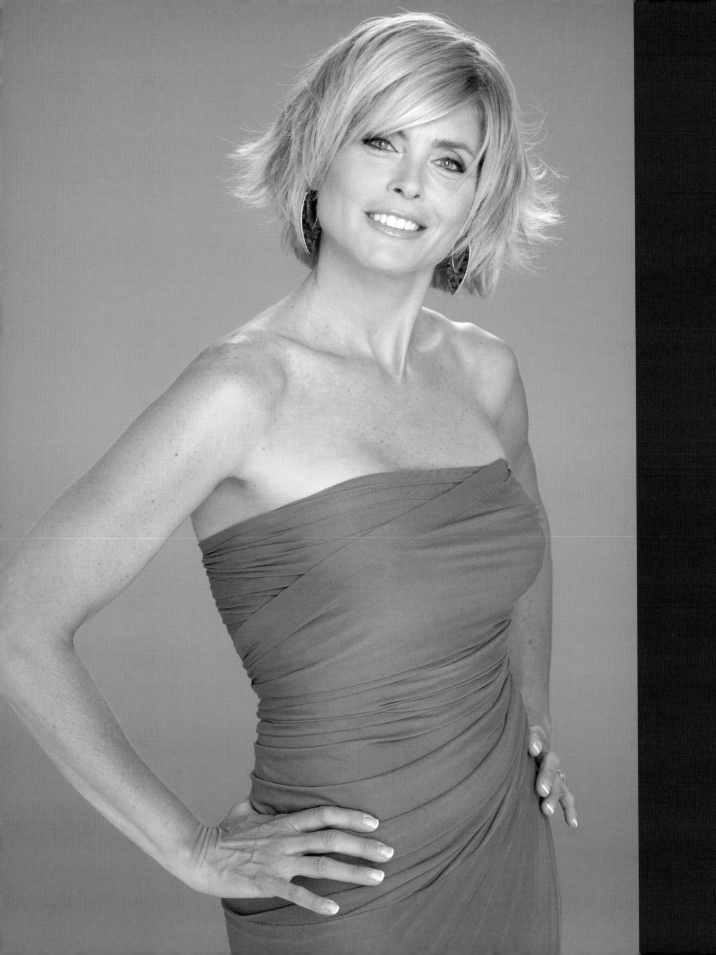

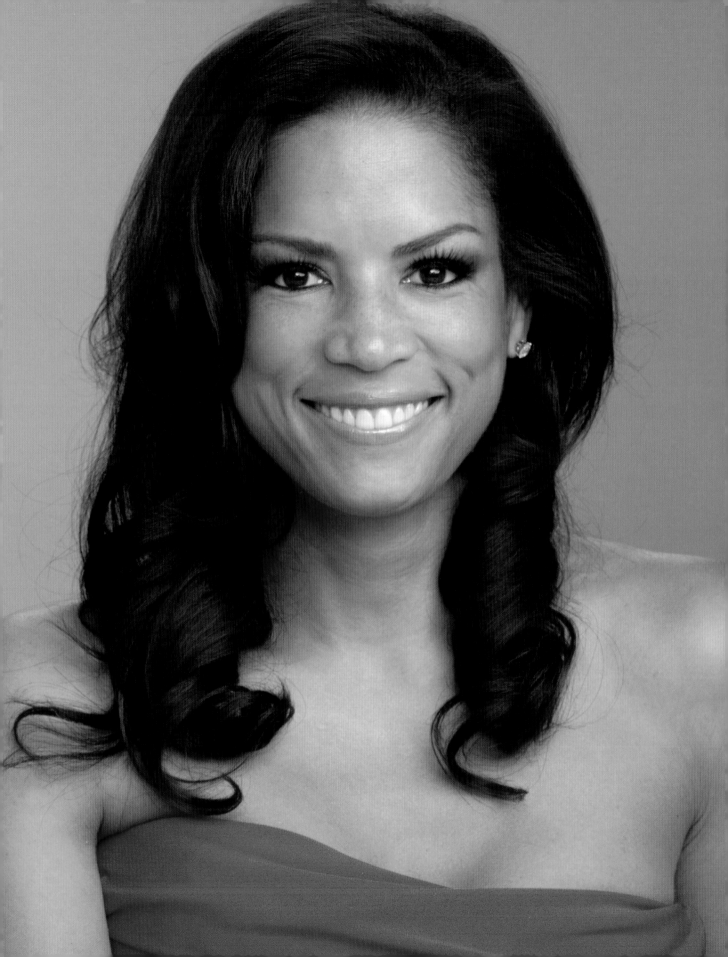

CHAPTER SEVEN

CRACKING THE MAKEUP CODE

Here are the secrets of a top beauty editor and celebrity makeup artist:

Our generation really lucked out. Our timing is impeccable. Makeup and skincare have changed in a big way during the last couple of decades and all for the better—just in time for us to reap the benefits now. Recent major improvements in texture mean we can wear real color, definition, and coverage in a comfortable, modern way. Sandy and I ended every makeup lesson chapter of this book with product suggestions and sprinkled more product mentions throughout others. Now we'll explain our choices and let you in on the secrets behind the faces you see in magazines, ads, commercials, TV, movies—and on the street.

Veronica Webb

Staying current when it comes to products is part of the daily job for a beauty editor and makeup artist. We need to know what's new and what's best and they aren't always the same thing. Are you surprised?

Why we recommend certain products

Beauty is a business and competition between brands is fierce. The number and speed of new product launches in the makeup arena is overwhelming for consumers of every age, but specifically for women our age, who have seen and worn it all. Sandy and I sample and test thousands of makeup products every year, but not many make our favorites list. Here's why: a lot of products are better suited to teens and younger women. They may be too trendy, too dry, too shiny, too glittery, too garish, too girly, or downright ineffective for us. Others don't make the cut because they don't meet our expectations in terms of color, texture, performance, or application.

When it comes to new products, we look for those that technology has improved in terms of texture and color. We're all for upgrading the basics and making application easier. Without technology we would not have high-density eye pencils, buildable sheer foundations, or silky, light, high-pigment lipsticks.

You'll notice we have a fondness for certain brands and an absence of others on our list. Don't feel you have to buy everything new and start all over again. Our purpose is to not give you a laundry list of must-haves, but suggestions to guide you in adding to, updating, or upgrading your makeup kit. Use these as a starting point and check them out by testing them in-store to get an idea of why they rate so highly with us. You may have your own brand preferences or products you love. That's fine too. For some of you, Sandy's makeup lessons and our advice can show you how to maximize the benefits of the makeup you already own. It may be all you need.

Our "loves" are a mix of new and simply amazing basics that have stuck around because they're just so good, always available, and we know they work.

What's the best way to shop for makeup? Online? Department store? Drugstore?

Beauty moves fast in this age of instant Internet information. Public relations teams, the news-breaking branch of cosmetic companies, have speeded up the process of getting news to consumers. Brand websites often provide immediate purchase online or a link to a beauty retail website. Social media like Facebook and Twitter and beauty bloggers have accelerated access to new products way beyond the traditional format of beauty magazines and print advertising with their three-month lead time. Viral venues are giving brands the opportunity to get instant feedback from makeup users too. Consumers can submit questions or give input on products themselves. The makeup shopper has become a powerful voice in the behind-the-scenes decision-making process of every cosmetic company.

It's not just about price or status anymore—makeup has become as much about personal style as fashion is.

Everyone knows women cross-shop for everything, including makeup. You might buy a Lancôme foundation at Nordstrom, stop at Duane Reade for Maybelline mascara, re-order Bobbi Brown concealer online, and dash into Sephora to try new Stila eye shadows—all in the same day.

If you love shopping online:

This eliminates two intimidating aspects of makeup shopping. You don't actually have to deal with a live human beauty advisor (unless you choose to), and you're not on a schedule. You can take as long as you like to make up your mind and there's no pressure to buy. You can go back and forth between brands in seconds, put items on hold in your virtual cart, and check out lipsticks at 2AM wearing your PJs or during a five-minute break at work.

Online shoppers get special offers and discounts and receive e-mail alerts about new products or promotions. There are brand site application videos complete with how-to steps, shade and texture guides, real shopper reviews of products, and interactive Q+As with beauty pros when you have a question. One that we hear often is: Are older women who are used to in-store shopping doing their beauty buying online? Yes, they are. This new way of shopping appeals to the new kind of 40+ woman, who dresses in a more youthful way, lives online, and likes the competitive edge of staying up to the minute in every way.

I love browsing online retailers like beauty.com, sephora.com, and brand-specific sites. It's my guilty pleasure as I graze through product reviews and ratings by customers, write my own critiques, and chat online with beauty advisors about specific products. Online color charts for makeup have come a long way and are much more shade-accurate—they practically jump off the page.

I also love the way some sites, like sephora.com, add exact shade and texture details in copy that help refine your search. For example, scrolling through the Laura Mercier Eye Colour shadows you see the shade Baroque and get the details, sateen/peachy gold shimmer, and for Morning Dew you are told it's a matte/light neutral pink. If you're deciding between two peach shadows at bobbibrown.com you learn that Seashell Shimmer Wash Eye Shadow is a medium golden peach and Champagne is a light golden peach. At beauty.com and its sister site, drugstore.com, you can cross-shop online for high and low brands in one virtual shopping bag. So you can get a NARS blush and Maybelline mascara with one checkout.

I shop online to reorder products I already know. But for me, nothing beats testing and trying new makeup live and in person in a store setting! However, I'm getting more and more comfortable and knowledgeable shopping online. It's so convenient.

If you love buying makeup at department stores:

Make department store shopping an opportunity to find a one-on-one beauty advisor or resident makeup artist (found more and more at counters full-time now). Pick a specific brand or two and establish a rapport. You'll get calls, emails, or personal notes reminding you about special workshops, promotions, and product launches. You can request free makeup lessons or mini-makeovers. If you're just browsing and don't intend to actually buy, ask if they have the time since these advisors work on commission. You can even get your makeup touched up en-route to a party or meeting!

 Department store makeup counters are excellent sources for improving your makeup skills or getting assistance with shade and texture selection. You might want to bring in your own makeup kit and show the beauty advisor or makeup artist what you've been using. She can help you integrate fresh updates into your existing makeup and suggest alternatives for products that are no longer working.

It's also a great opportunity to take advantage of free samples, which are generously offered. The return policy on the products you pick up here is easy if it does not perform as expected. Sticking with big-name brands is great for women who get a confidence boost from a brand they trust and know works for them. For the kind of woman who wears Michael Kors or Theory because they never miss for her, Lancôme, Estée Lauder, Chanel, or Bobbi Brown will provide the same easy one-stop solution.

 As a makeup pro, all I want is privacy to just look and test without having to explain anything. The reason is that I'm not looking and buying for myself but for my clients, who have a huge range of skin tones, and issues that are very different from my own. I want to be left on my own to browse when I shop without having to explain why.

For non-pros, counter beauty advisors and makeup artists provide the perfect opportunity to help you find the right foundation or explain differences in textures and shades. Unless you are naturally gifted at makeup application, you will benefit from their instruction.

If you love drugstores and mass retailer shopping:

You know a bargain when you see one. Savvy drugstore beauty shoppers see past the packaging and walls of products to the contemporary technology, shades, and textures that are driving these brands now. Lots of luxury brands get ideas from small, niche, or low-cost brands. It's how the whole mineral makeup trend began. Remember that the cardboard and plastic packaging gets tossed and it's the product that does the trick.

 Go online first for more product info before stepping foot in the store. For example, the L'Oréal Paris site (lorealparisusa.com) makes it easy for women who want to transition from a high-end department store brand or even another low-cost drugstore foundation. Just click on the Beauty Matchmaker filter and then click on the pull-downs to get your current brand and shade matched to a L'Oréal Paris one. When I tested it for examples of low-cost swaps, the site matched my Chanel Lift Lumière in Ivoire with L'Oréal Visible Lift in Nude Beige, and my Bobbi Brown Skin Foundation in Sand 2 with L'Oréal True Match Roller in W3 Nude Beige. If you decide to buy the alternative, there's a link to an online retailer, like drugstore.com. I wish every department store beauty site suggested brand options for similar shades and textures in every product.

Another site that offers advice is CoverGirl (covergirl.com), with its ColorMatch system that personalizes product selections based on your eyes, hair color, skin tone, and most flattering fashion colors.

 I browse drugstores too. Sometimes I come up with amazing finds such as makeup wipes. I found them in the late 1980s—years before they were sold in department stores. I get my pointy Q-tips there and Almay liquid liner.

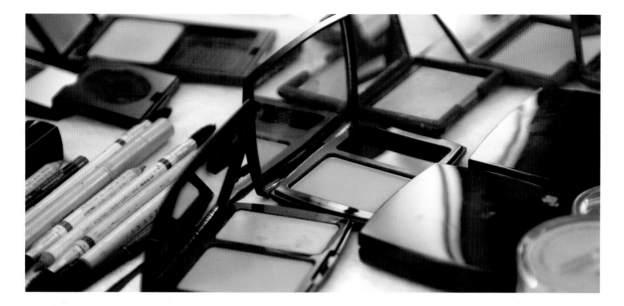

If you love Sephora:

Who doesn't? The Sephora do-it-yourself experience and mix of top and niche brands is hard to pass up. The typical Sephora shopper has a high aesthetic and knows what's new and how she likes her makeup to look. She also likes the set up, the mirrors, cleansers, wipes, and disposable applicators that make the shopping experience easy, hygienic, and personal.

Sandy says: If you like to play around with makeup and don't want anyone or anything coming between you and the product, Sephora is your dream store. The self-service approach, easy-to-navigate aisles with no counters, and super-organized layout of product by brand at eye level makes makeup shopping like being a kid in a candy store. You can try on as many products and brands at a time as you like with no "help" unless desired and no pressure to buy.

Lois says: It's easy to roam from Laura Mercier to Make Up For Ever to Guerlain, so you can try a Laura Mercier Foundation with a Guerlain bronzer or a Lancôme shadow with a NARS liner. If you live in a city with a Sephora store (there are more than two hundred locations in the US and Canada)—lucky you.

Veronica Webb

"I've worked hard to become who and what I am—spiritually, mentally, emotionally, and physically. My favorite things in life are beauty and discipline. You have to stick to what's good for you, what works for you. I'm a minimalist, but an extremist. Having children helped me a lot; your time for yourself is limited, so you have to be efficient. In beauty and style you always have pack leaders, type-A personalities who are always ahead of the curve or right on the curve, like Mrs. Obama and her drive for health and fitness in this country. It's great to see a substantial change in diversity of imagery in the beauty industry now. There's a wider range of ages, ethnicities, and sexual orientation seen in the media. For myself, I like a split between what's good for you and what's totally natural. Makeup's as simple as a lash, a line, concealer, and a little shimmer."

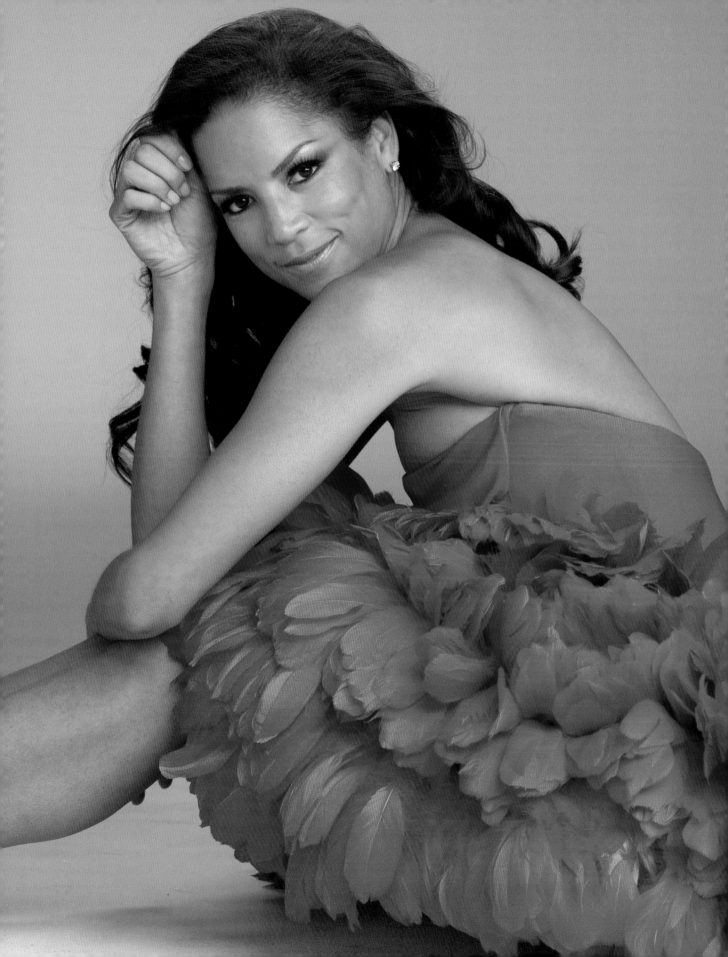

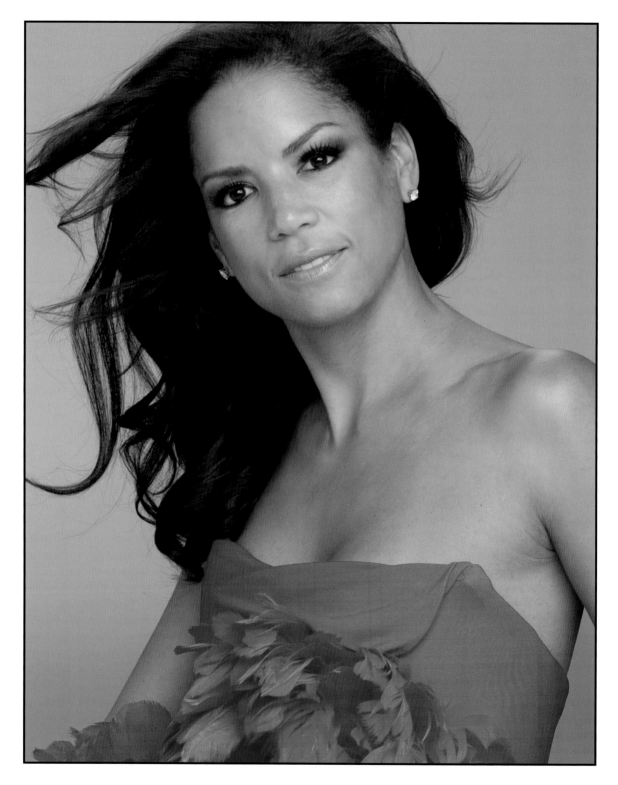

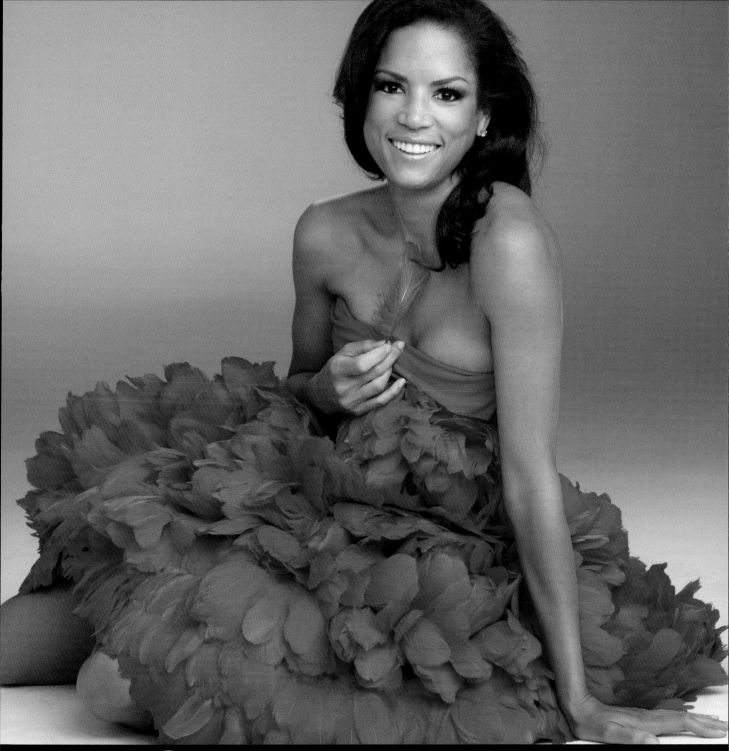

A red dress doesn't need a red lip. Put the focus on your eyes.

Why makeup credited to magazine photos often does not look that way in real life.

Makeup alone isn't responsible for the fabulous older faces in magazine photos and ads. You're looking at basically beautiful people altered by lighting. Remember that hair pros, editors, and stylists have also toiled for hours to get the look right. And then there is the miracle of Photoshop to make double chins and turkey necks vanish, soften expression lines, and brighten teeth. We've seen ordinary faces turn extraordinary with lighting and post-shoot retouching. In magazines and advertising it's this "virtual surgery" on lines, sags, spots, and bags that makes you wonder why you don't look that way. Why do you think paparazzi love to get those no-makeup daylight shots of stars? At home, it's just you and your 10X mirror and the mileage on your face. Use it to get your detail work done and then stand back! You won't ever achieve what happens with retouching, so get real.

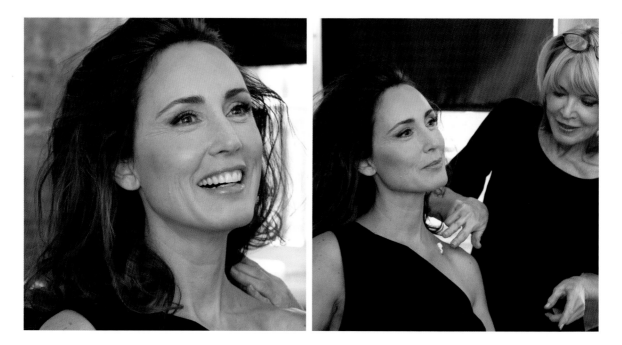

When a makeup artist applies makeup on a shoot the end result is a true work-in-progress. Actually, it's often how makeup trends start. In the process of layering and blending, brands are often mixed and shades or textures are created that don't exist as a single product. As a result, the makeup you see credited (sometimes months later) is often a simulation of the actual products used. The products suggested by magazines allow readers to get a similar look with the newest products available.

There's retouching going on. Highlights are added to emphasize bone structure, colors are altered in Photoshop, pores and lines are erased, smudges and smears are cleaned up, lashes are added, lips and eyes are made bigger. Use these images to get inspired, but buy products that honestly work for you.

The point is: don't get caught up in buying a cosmetic simply because it looked great on a celebrity in an ad or magazine—even if they are over forty.

Makeup pros come to shoots with a huge and often diverse kit of makeup because they never know what the challenges of the day will bring. They can't predict the exact look, skin condition, or particular needs of a model or celebrity in advance. They don't know what the lighting will be like or even whether the shoot will be in black and white or color. They don't know exactly what the client/photographer/creative director/editor will require.

The cost of looking good

The prices of drugstore and department store makeup have gone up considerably since we were all in our twenties and thirties, and the economic arguments for that escalation are compelling. Improvements cost more whether the change is in drugstore mascara or a luxury brand lipstick. Sometimes a price jump is due to new technology, sometimes new ingredients, and sometimes it's caused by a better delivery system or packaging innovation.

Research and development teams within every makeup brand are constantly seeking ways to improve their best sellers and eliminate performance problems. Some products are fads that come and go in a season. Some products or lines within a brand stay, but the colors change or are edited. In drugstore beauty, the word "new" on the package is a shout to shoppers to pay attention. Give us a guess-timate. How much do you think you've spent on makeup you never wore or regretted buying? We bet it's thousands.

Buying new makeup has always been a slightly risky venture but there's an element of excitement and reward we look forward to in the end. If you've become jaded, bored, or fed up with makeup shopping it's time to bring back the thrill.

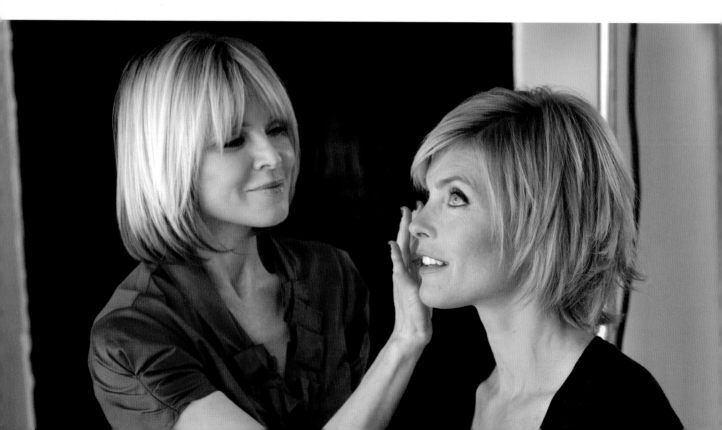

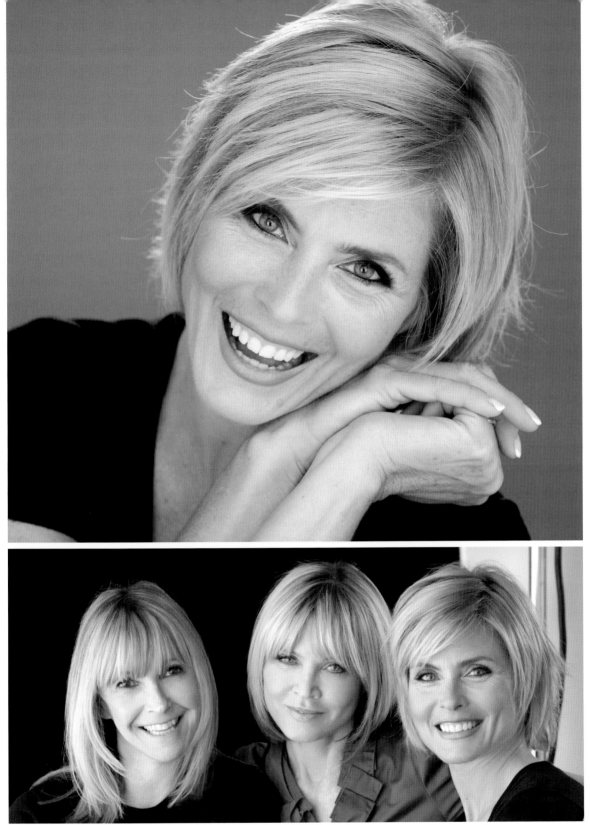

Lois, Sandy, and Kim—we strive to stay contemporary to look our best.

6 Beauty Tips that Change Everything

1   **All makeup is not created equal.** That old eye pencil story about "they all come from the same two factories" is just an old story.

2   **Shop high and low. It's a myth that expensive is always better.** Once upon a long time ago, say back to the '80s, this was absolutely true. But things have changed. First of all scientists, researchers, and teams of dermatologists and marketers working behind the scenes in cosmetic company labs have democratized beauty. They've closed the gap between department store and drugstore brands, especially in skincare. Now whether your moisturizer/wrinkle cream costs $20 or $200, it's the scientific evidence, lab technology, and specific ingredients that make the difference in your skin. And whether your foundation costs $13.99 or $55, it's often the texture, shade, and research behind it that make the difference in the quality.

If you want the smartest buy for less, stick to one of the big global beauty giants, like the L'Oréal Group, Procter & Gamble, or Beiersdorf, which have high and low brands within their companies. They have the resources and money to keep all their brands on the cutting edge and enable their low-cost brands to keep pace with their high-end sisters.

Did you know, for example, that L'Oréal owns the drugstore brands L'Oréal Paris and Maybelline, specialty pharmacy brands Vichy and La Roche-Posay, SkinCeuticals, Kiehl's—and the luxury brands Lancôme, Giorgio Armani Beauty, and Yves Saint Laurent Beauty? Procter & Gamble owns Olay, CoverGirl, and also the expensive SK-II. Beiersdorf owns Nivea, Eucerin, and the ultra-costly La Prairie!

OK, you ask—if drugstore is so great why should I ever spend more? Because some pricey makeup and skincare absolutely fulfill their claims, so let's not pretend they don't. Say you have fallen in love with an Yves Saint Laurent Rouge Volupté Lipstick—if you adore the texture and color, it makes your lips feel gorgeous, and most of all you can afford it, why argue with success? But if fancy packaging is what ensnares you, don't get caught up in the high price tag unless what's inside does the trick. Once it's on your face no one knows what it is anyway. There are so many no-name brands out there now, lots of unreliable junk being hyped on the Internet, and small niche brands that have one- or two-star products. If you want quality skip these in favor of brands with a reputation for customer service and quality.

3 Stop trying so hard to hide the fact that you wear makeup.
It's crazy when you are wearing foundation, concealer, blush, eyeliner, and lipstick to pretend you're not. Honestly, at this age you're not fooling anyone into thinking you sprang out of bed that way.

Why not simply go for it? Find the right shades and textures. Stick to warm earthy neutrals that won't scream "fakery," and follow Sandy's makeup lessons. You probably wear a body shaper and underwire bra, jeans with a little stretch in them, longer tees with sleeves, so what's the problem? When makeup is right it only makes you look better, smarter, more confident.

4 Satisfy your urge for color in small doses.
We all have a fashion moment when things go awry. Have you ever come home with a red sheath dress and a pink Prada satchel when you really need a tailored gray skirt and a sleek black bag for work?

We have. It's that moment when you tell your colorist to brighten up your highlights to gold, or ask your manicurist for violet instead of Essie Ballet Slippers. A little color splurge now and then can make you happy without jeopardizing your integrity as a class act. Never forget you're a black-belt shopper with over twenty years experience as your own personal stylist and fashion therapist. Be as strategic with makeup as you are with clothes but have fun too. You only need one item to do it.

5 **"De-aging" makeup is still makeup first.** This well-meaning category can be frustrating because not every woman 40+ has the same issues. Some of us have dry, thin skin; others have oily, thicker skin, big pores, blackheads, breakouts; some have pigmentation issues; and others are bothered by lines and creases. Some of us have hard-to-match skin tones; some are so dark or so pale or blotchy that they have never found a true foundation color match. Some of us have skin that gobbles up makeup quickly; others have skin that rejects makeup. We may all be aging, but we're doing it at our own pace and in a very personal way.

Have you ever heard a woman say, "I look older wearing makeup?" Any woman that says so is not applying it correctly. For instance, the difference between a beautiful soft brow and an incorrectly shaped and drawn in brow could be a difference in years. Get hands-on help if you need it by asking questions of a beauty pro. Find someone who can see *you* and not a customer. Trust us, it can happen and you will benefit from instruction.

6 **Ask yourself: Do I look amazing? Is this product fantastic on me or am I blinded by the color, label, hype, or packaging?** Give potential makeup a test-drive on the back of your hand or face (if you can actually have an in-store makeup artist apply it), take a break, and come back a half hour or an hour later to see if you still feel the same way.

If you're really interested in buying makeup have it applied to see what it looks like first. If you can't have it applied, ask questions to find out if the product's meant for your skin type and age.

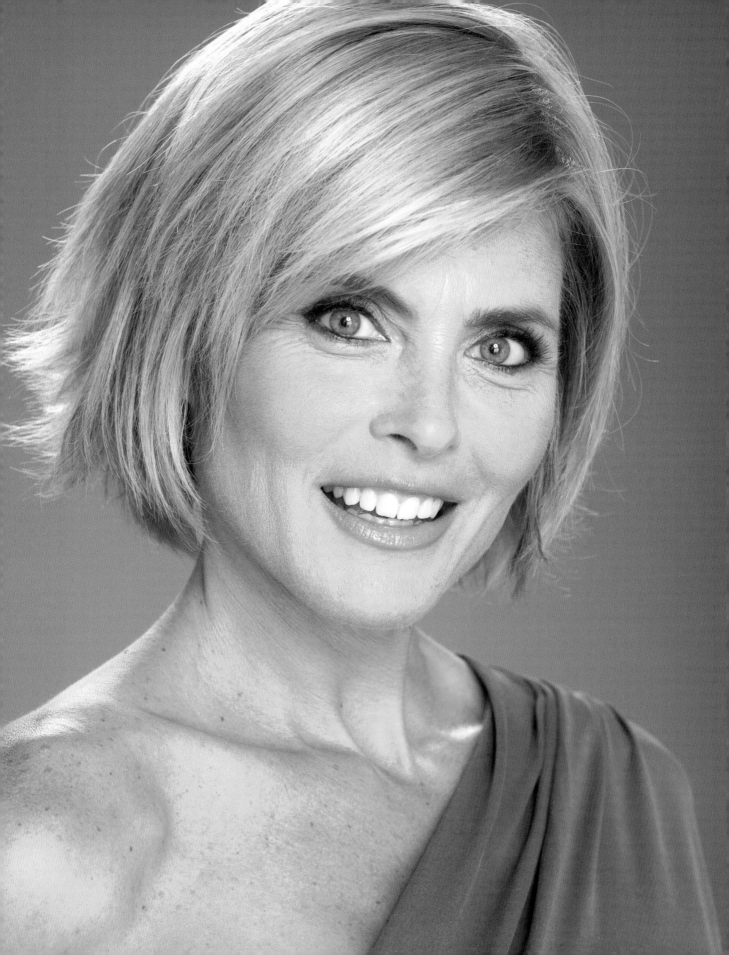

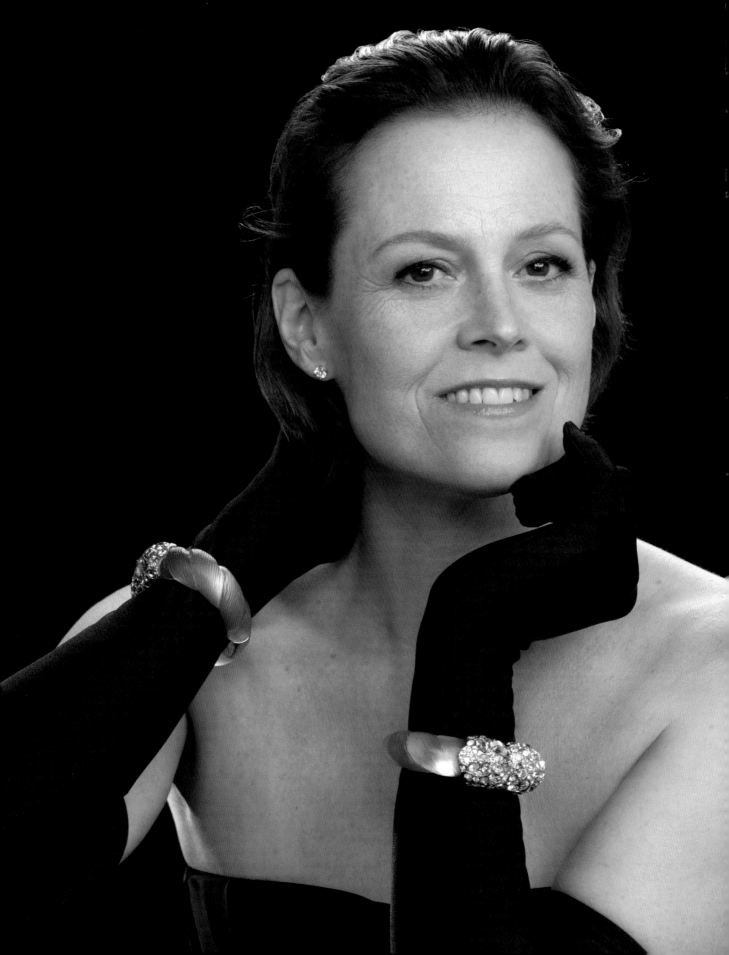

Sigourney Weaver

"My mother's friends were the most chic and fun group of women—they loved life, loved their experiences. They always looked great and just went ahead and lived. They didn't obsess about age and every little line. I learned a lot from them. If I put makeup on I want to look like I'm wearing makeup, but I do think I look better with less makeup. When I'm on my own, I curl my lashes and do some blush and eyebrows. I like seeing the blood under the skin, staying fresh and light.

I think older women are incredibly beautiful, especially women who look interesting—women who allow themselves to go gray. That over-maintained look, the frozen, straight-off-the-designer runway look, is very aging. After fifty we've put in our time, we've raised a family, run businesses, worked, and we have so much verve and life force in us. It's not about perfection; it's about taking good care of your skin, eating correctly, exercising, and having energy and passion for life. At sixty, it's not time to stay the same— it's time to explode. Don't ever be finished."

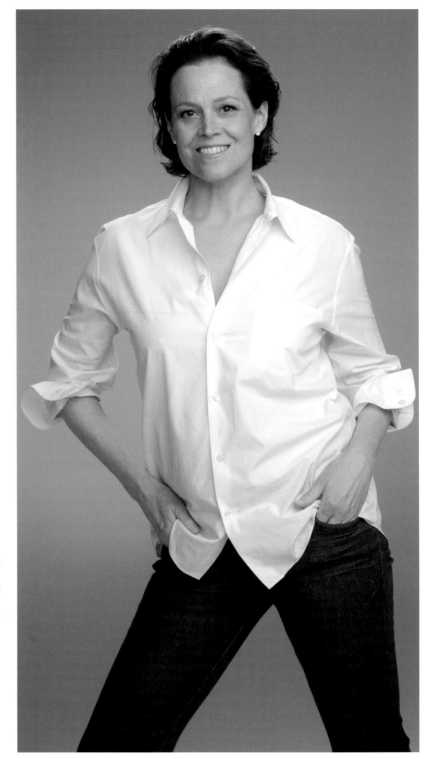

 Going from jeans to black tie can be as simple as applying a stronger lip color.

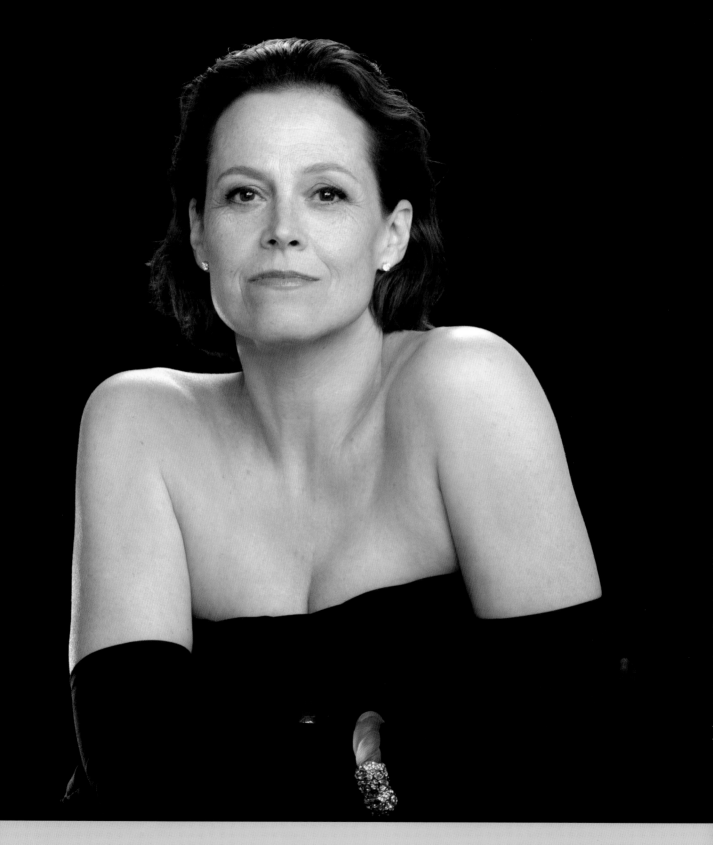

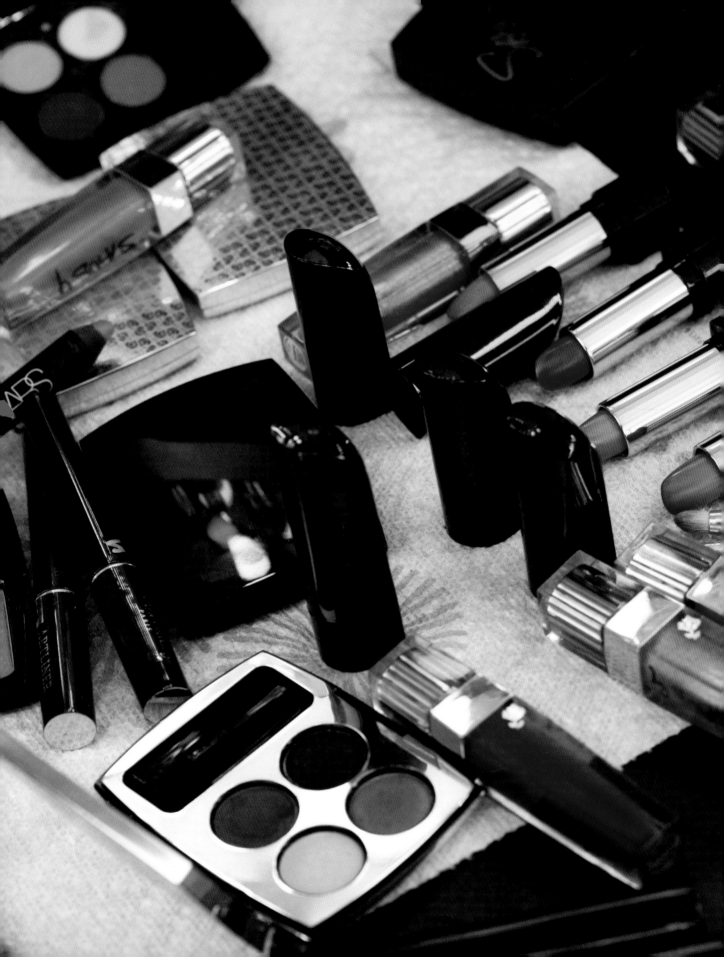

The To-Do List
Sandy's Steps To Makeup Confidence

We thought we'd close with a checklist of all the steps it takes to do your entire face in full makeup. Here's the proof—Sandy herself in a before, after, and everything that goes in between makeup session. Use these pages as a quick reminder of what, when, where, and how. You may want to edit or eliminate steps to suit your own preferences or needs on a particular day.

Before

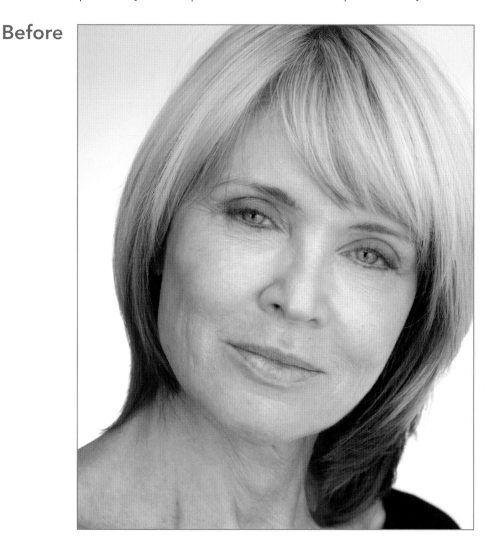

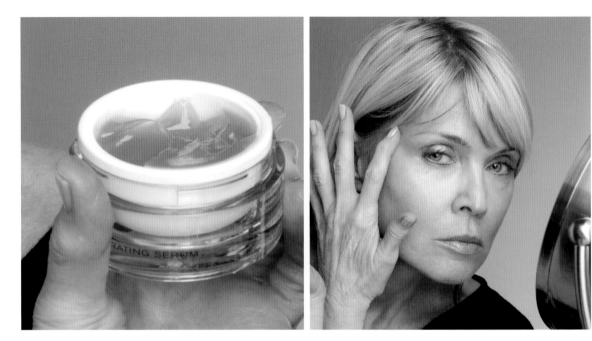

1. First, prepare the face with moisturizer and sun protection or serum.

2. Apply primer to the eyelid.

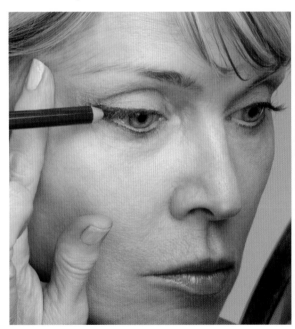

3. Pencil on black or dark brown liner. Thicken the line at the outer end.

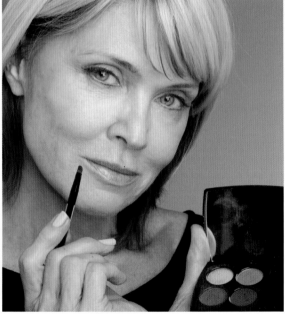

4. Select your eye shadow kit. It should include retrace shadow liner, lid shadow, and hollow shadow.

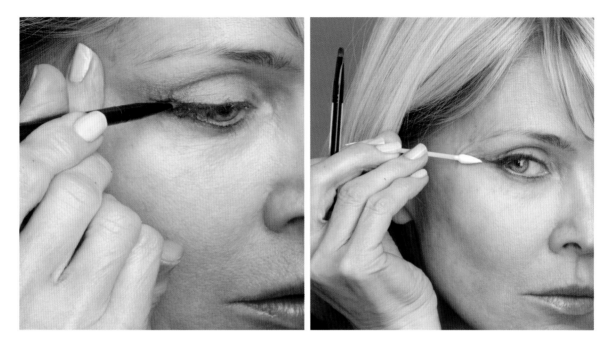

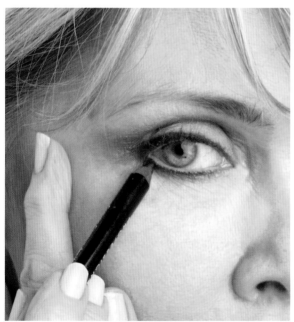

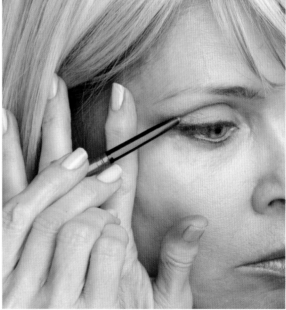

5. Re-line over the pencil with matching powder shadow using a firm liner brush.

6. Kick the line up with a cotton swab.

7. Line lower lids with pencil. Start at the outer corner and work your way in. Don't connect with the upper line.

8. Contour the eye hollow with neutral pencil. Blend with a shadow brush made for eye hollow in an upward direction.

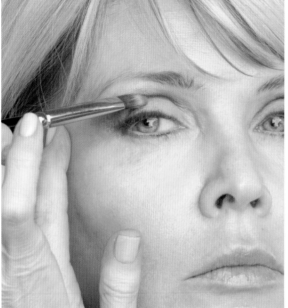

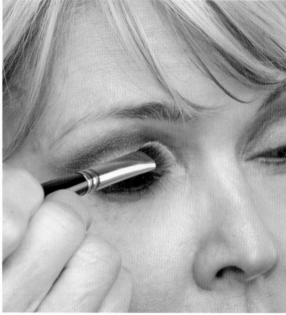

9. Retrace the hollow with complementary shadow.

10. Apply a light shadow to the lids.

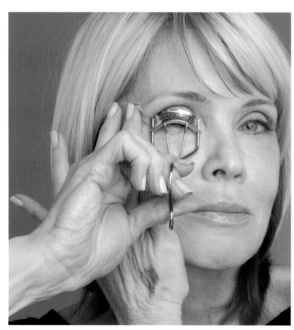

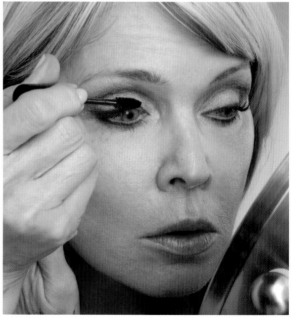

11. Cup lashes into the curler. Flick wrist up and curl.

12. Add black mascara on top lashes.

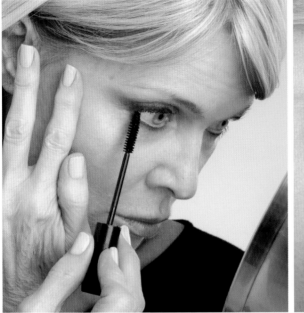

13. Add mascara to bottom lashes—hold wand vertically.

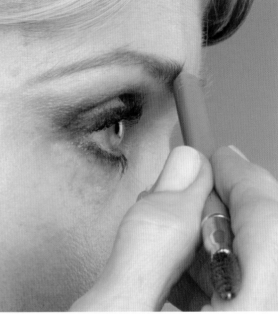

14. Extend brows and fill where necessary.

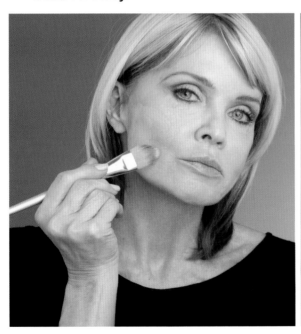

15. Brush on foundation; use the back of your hand as a palette.

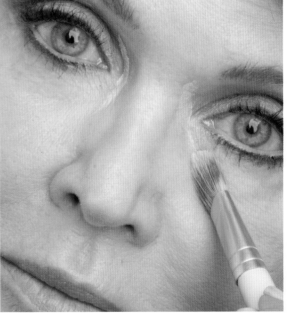

16. Brush on concealer where necessary.

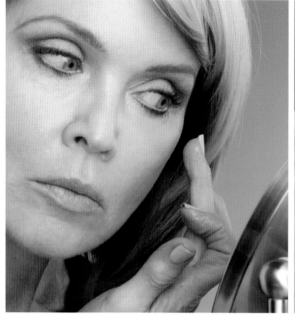

17. Apply blush high on the cheekbones.

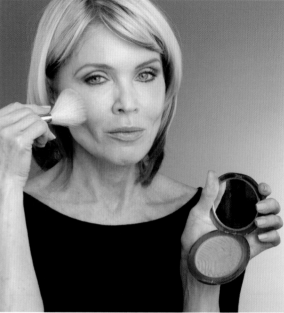

18. Add bronzing powder for extra glow in a C shape (optional).

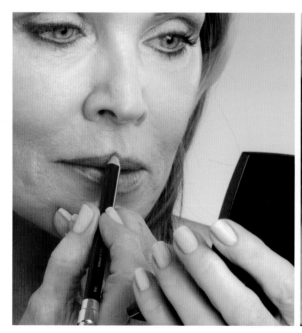

19. Correct lips with lip-toned pencil.

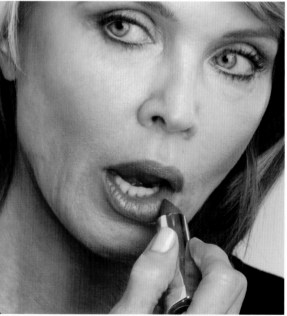

20. Add lipstick and gloss or do entire lip with lip pencil and gloss. Or, use lipstick alone.

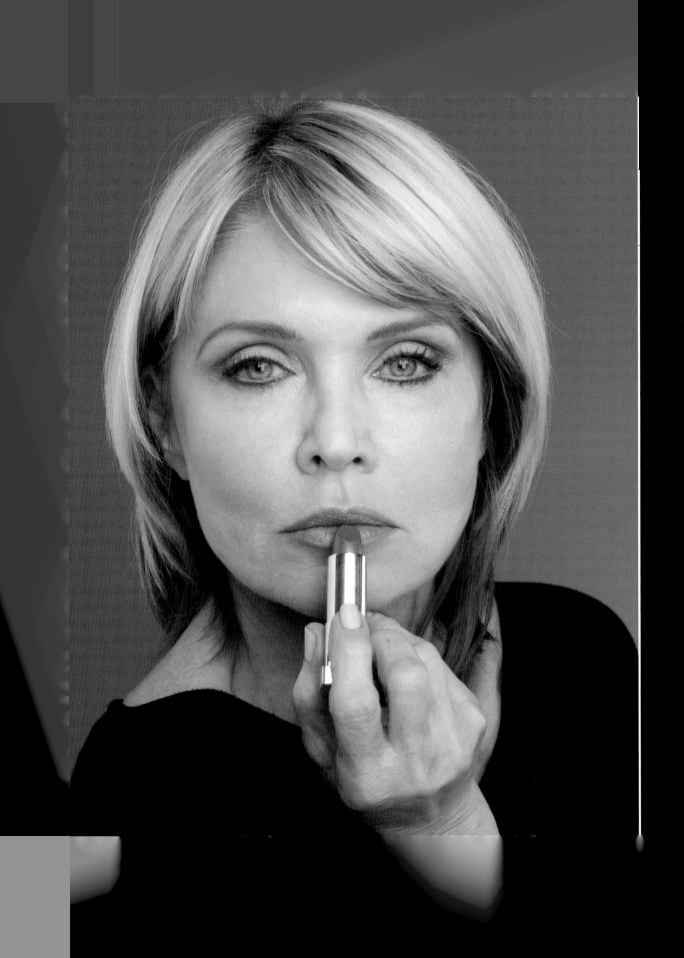

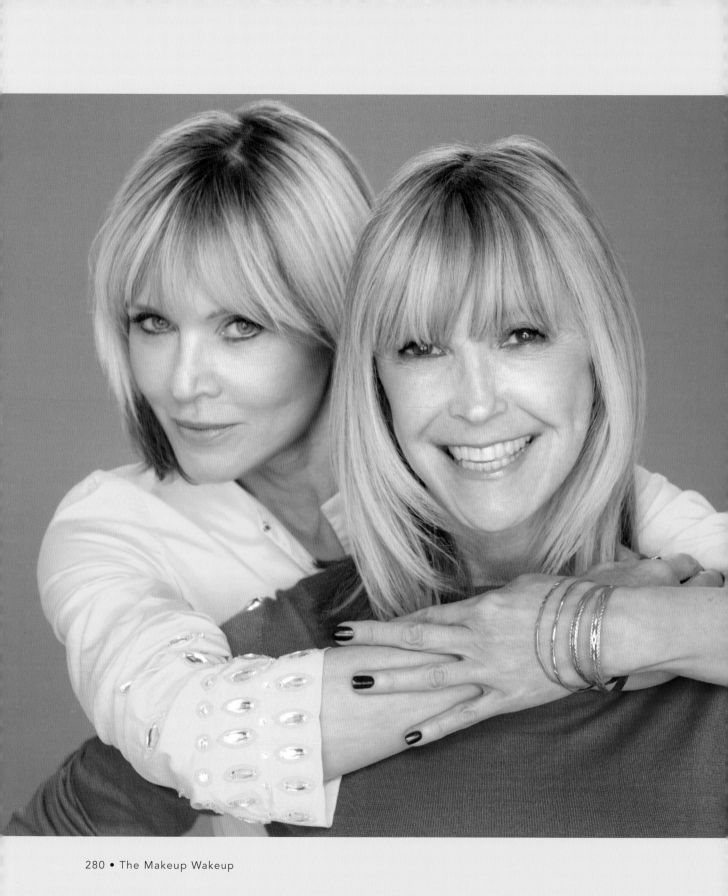

Thank You from SANDY + LOIS

To our extraordinary photographer, Michael Waring, who filled all our studio days with gorgeous lighting and extraordinary photos.

To Dr. Daniel Baker, Dr. Fredric Brandt, and Dr. Patricia Wexler, for sharing your knowledge and experience with us and our readers.

To The Girls—Kim Alexis, Carol Alt, Karen Bjornson, Alva Chinn, Nancy Donahue, Lauren Ezersky, Patti Hansen, Deborah Harry, Lana Ogilvie, Jane Powers, Joanne Russell, Cheryl Tiegs, Sigourney Weaver, Veronica Webb, Constance White, and Julie Wolfe . . . for being there for us and taking the time from all you do.

To Bette Midler, for reading this and writing a genuine, wonderful foreword with heart and soul—and for impromptu copy-editing skills.

To Jill Hattersley, assistant to Bette Midler, for magic scheduling and making things happen.

To **Sigourney Weaver,** for making a spectacular day for us.

To **Hannelies Hartman,** assistant to Sigourney Weaver.

To photographer **Jonathan Pushnik,** for photographing Ms. Midler for the foreword.

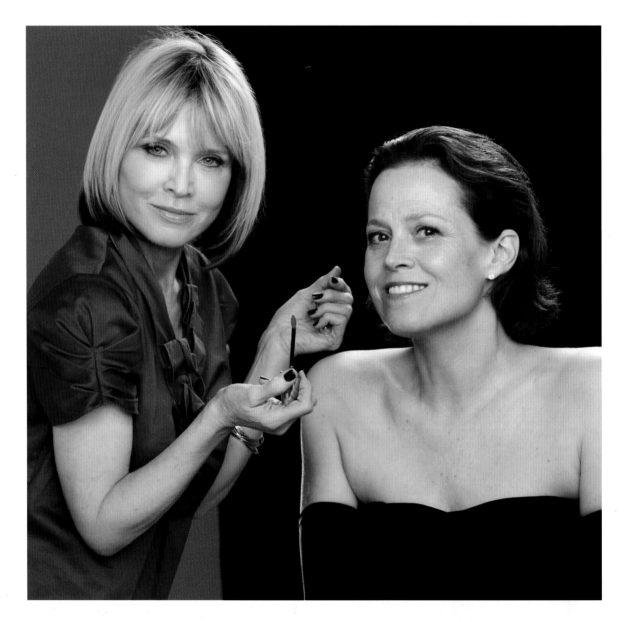

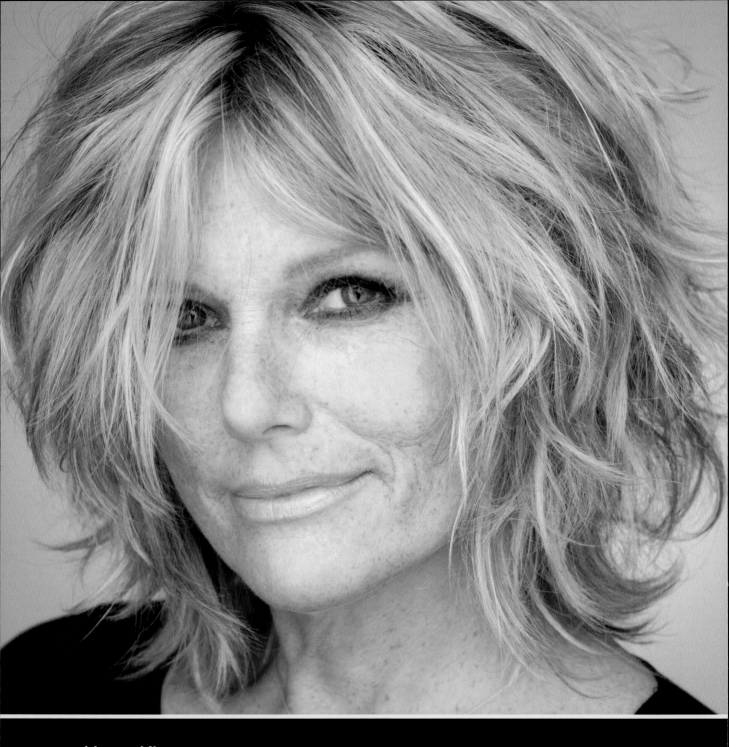

To **Harry King,** for hair on Nancy Donahue, Patti Hansen, and Alva Chinn.

To **Robert Lyon,** for hair on Lauren Ezersky, Constance White, Karen Bjornson, Cheryl Tiegs, and Joanne Russell.

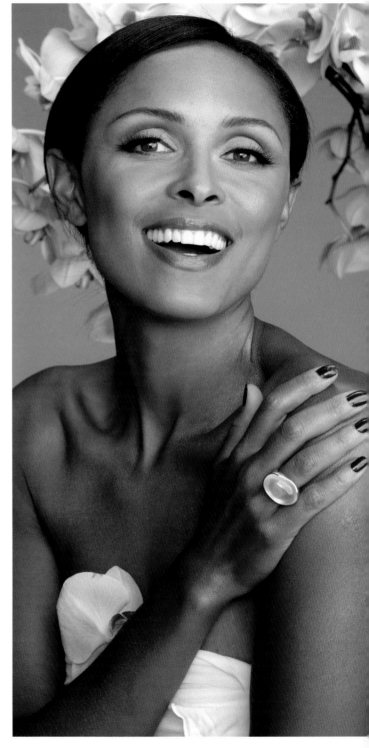

To **Felix Fischer** for hair on Julie Wolfe and Carol Alt.

To **Nelson Vercher,** of the Rita Hazan Salon, for hair on Lana Ogilvie and Veronica Webb.

To **Juan Carlos Maciques** and his assistant, **Christina Bosque,** of the Rita Hazan Salon, for Ms. Midler's hair.

To **Maury Hopson,** for hair on Sigourney Weaver.

To **Mitch Barry,** for hair on Kim Alexis and Jane Powers.

To **RoseAnn Singelton,** celebrity manicurist, for the nails on Lana Ogilvie.

To **Freddie Leiba,** for styling Constance White, Joanne Russell, and Karen Bjornson.

To **Bill Mullen,** for styling Deborah Harry and Carol Alt, and thanks to his assistant, **Mauricio Quezada.**

To **Aimee Galimidi,** for styling Julie Wolfe and Lana Ogilvie.

To **Jonny Lichtenstein,** for styling Bette Midler, Sigourney Weaver, Kim Alexis, and Jane Powers, and last-minute model skills.

To **Jordy Poon,** for makeup assistance, styling, and cat wrangling.

To **Oslyn Holder,** for makeup assistance.

To **Natalie DiStefano,** for makeup on Lois Joy Johnson and assistance to Sandy.

To **Deborah Pagani Jewelry,** for jewelry on Jane Powers, Lana Ogilvie, Carol Alt, and Kim Alexis.

To everyone at **Runner Collective,** including **Tracy Boychuk, Tina Ibanez, Elizabeth Romanazzi,** and **Brett Kilroe.**

To everyone at **Shoot Digital,** for being so generous and wonderful and making our studio days easy, including **Randy Mitev, Cassidy Parker, Brad Jamieson, Tony Lord, Joanna Hoepner, Peter Rainis,** and **Hector Tirado.**

To **Michael Waring's** photo assistants, **Joe Leonard, Robert Massman, Evan Lee,** and **Elise Bruccoliere,** for on-set support.

To **Alexander Yerks** and **Jim Geist** for digital tech help.

To **Fred Blake** at **Fotocare Rental.**

To **Noz,** for catering.

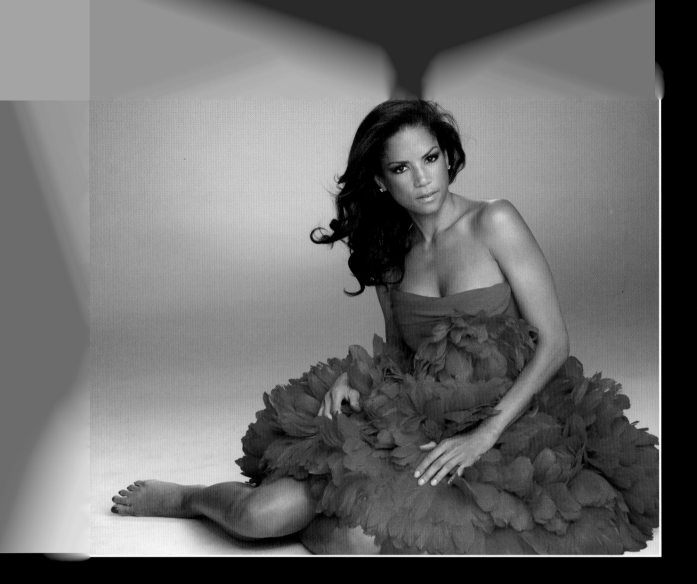

To **Running Press**, our editor, **Cindy De La Hoz,** and our book designer **Corinda Cook,** for making this book a reality.

To **Kerry Diamond** at Lancôme, for sharing our vision for *The Makeup Wakeup*.

To **Vanessa Dabich** for all her support.

To our brilliant and resilient literary agent, **Alice Martell.**

To **Patty Sicular** at **Ford Models,** for all your help.

To our color gurus, Brad Johns (Lois) and Rita Hazan (Sandy), for great quotes and making us look so good all year round.

To the P.R. Team at Saks Fifth Avenue, for contributing the clothes for Cheryl Tiegs, Sigourney Weaver, Jane Powers, and Kim Alexis.

To Irina Shabayeva, for Veronica Webb's dress.

To Zeze Flowers, for the gorgeous flowers, and Trixie the cat.

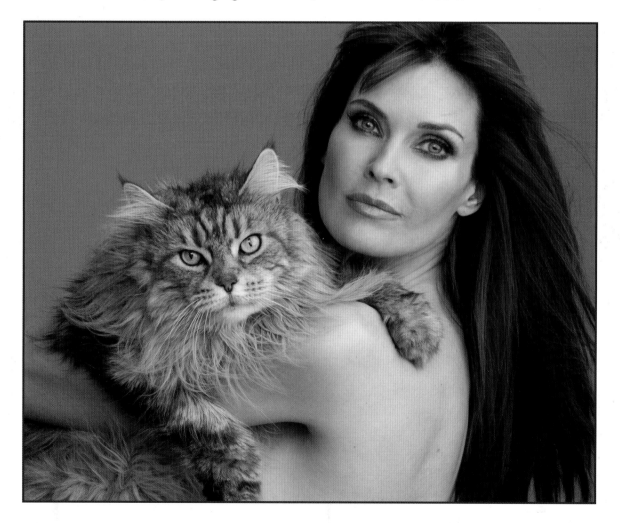

To Lois's BFFs,
**Charla Krupp,
Marilyn Glass,**
and **Gloria Appel,**
for enthusiasm, love, and
support always, all the time.

To Sandy's BFFs
Sherry Lynn
(my gorgeous friend
and client) and
Linda Ramone
(whose styling tips
are always appreciated).

To Lois's daughters,
Jennifer Jolie and
Alexandra Jade
for keeping the family
beauty tradition going.

And to Sandy's newlywed
sister, **Susan Brint.**
We agree on one thing
only, "It's never too late."

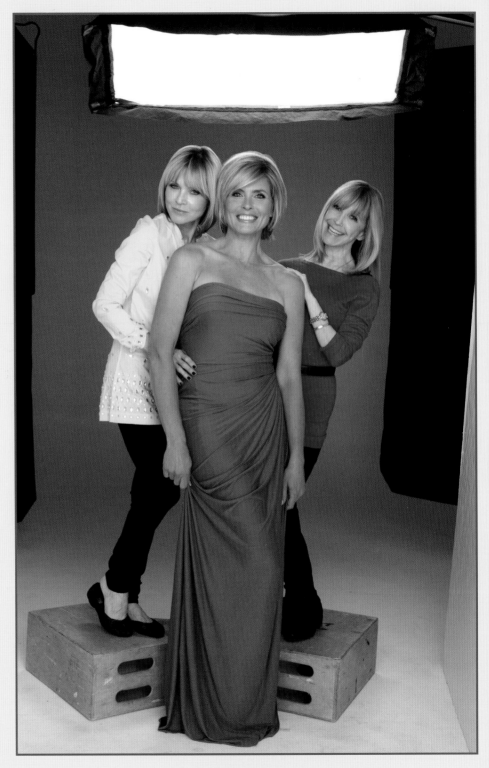